Whether you are one of the millions who takes antidepressants or a patient's concerned family member or
loved one, this invaluable guide gives you the most up-to-
date information and tells you everything you need to
know about:

- The pros and cons of taking an antidepressant, anti-
anxiety agent, or hypnotic
- Which medications can be taken in combination with
others
- Side effects—and how to manage them
- How to get off your drugs safely
- What to do if your last drug failed
- What therapy and drugs can do together
- What is blocking your cure

"Much wise advice, to both patients and their helpers,
from an experienced and honest clinician."
—Leston Havens, M.D., professor of psychiatry,
Harvard Medical School

WILLIAM S. APPLETON, M.D., is a psychiatrist who has been
in private practice for forty years. He is the author of several books on psychiatric drugs written for professionals
as well as general readers. He is a member of the Harvard
Medical School faculty, and lives in Cambridge, Massachusetts.

Other Books by William Appleton, M.D.

Practical Clinical Psychopharmacology, 3rd Edition
The Fifth Psychoactive Drug Usage Guide

THE NEW ANTIDEPRESSANTS AND ANTIANXIETIES

WHAT YOU NEED TO KNOW ABOUT ZOLOFT, PAXIL, WELLBUTRIN, EFFEXOR, CLONAZEPAM, AMBIEN, AND MORE

William S. Appleton, M.D.

Previously published as
Prozac and the New Antidepressants

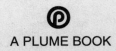

A PLUME BOOK

Every effort has been made to ensure that the information contained in this book is complete and accurate. However, neither the publisher nor the author is engaged in rendering professional advice or services to the individual reader. The ideas, procedures, and suggestions contained in this book are not intended as a substitute for consulting with your physician. All matters regarding your health require medical supervision. Neither the author nor the publisher shall be liable or responsible for any loss or damage allegedly arising from any information or suggestion in this book.

PLUME
Published by the Penguin Group
Penguin Group (USA) Inc., 375 Hudson Street, New York, New York 10014, U.S.A.
Penguin Books Ltd, 80 Strand, London WC2R 0RL, England
Penguin Books Australia Ltd, 250 Camberwell Road, Camberwell, Victoria 3124, Australia
Penguin Books Canada Ltd, 10 Alcorn Avenue, Toronto, Ontario, Canada M4V 3B2
Penguin Books India (P) Ltd, 11 Community Centre, Panchsheel Park, New Delhi – 110 017, India
Penguin Books (NZ), cnr Airborne and Rosedale Roads, Albany, Auckland 1310, New Zealand
Penguin Books (South Africa) (Pty) Ltd, 24 Sturdee Avenue, Rosebank, Johannesburg 2196, South Africa

Penguin Books Ltd, Registered Offices: 80 Strand, London WC2R 0RL, England

First published by Plume, a member of Penguin Group (USA) Inc., as *Prozac and the New Antidepressants*

First Printing, January 1997
First Printing (Revised Edition), January 2000
First Printing (Second Revised Edition), October 2004
10 9 8 7 6 5 4 3 2

 REGISTERED TRADEMARK—MARCA REGISTRADA

CIP data is available.
ISBN 0-452-28515-1

Printed in the United States of America
Set in New Baskerville
Designed by Leonard Telesca

To the memories of Gerald L. Klerman, M.D., and Elvin Semrad, M.D. Dr. Klerman taught me the importance of the precise description of psychiatric conditions, which enables mental health practitioners to communicate with one another, focuses research, and helps in evaluating treatments. Dr. Semrad believed the opposite, that "often when you get to know a patient they lose their diagnosis." Without Klerman's groupings, there can be no science, while the absence of Semrad's focus on the unique individual leaves no heart.

Contents

Acknowledgments

I wish to thank my editor, Gary Brozek, whose kind, firm hand guided me. Thanks also to Lindy Hess, my wife, whose help and encouragement sustain me. I am especially grateful to my colleagues at the Massachusetts Mental Health Center, who have taught me most of what I know about psychiatric drugs, psychotherapy, and taking care of patients. My patients have taught me the most, when I remember to keep my mind open and listen. What few answers we have in psychiatry lie in them, not in ourselves. My students try to keep me up-to-date as I attempt to help them apply their book knowledge to the human beings in their care. Thanks to Karen Wood for turning my handwriting into computer form.

Author's Note

The dosages and indications of the drugs in this book conform to the standards of the U.S. Food and Drug Administration and the practices of the general medical community. However, the usage of some of the medications in certain conditions may not have specific FDA approval. Because therapeutic standards continually change, it is necessary for readers to have their treatment supervised by a physician directly involved in their care.

Disclosure

For forty years I have been a psychopharmacologist and psychotherapist who has followed and tried to understand the findings of the neuroscientist and translate them into useful clinical practice. I have never taken a dollar from a drug company in the form of speaking honoraria or research support. There are very few experts in psychopharmacology—the study of the effects of drugs on mood, thinking, and behavior—who can make this claim. While I do not mean to imply that the overwhelming number of psychopharmacologists who have financial arrangements with one or many companies are tainted, I just wish to underline my own complete independence.

Introduction to the 2004 Edition

Many of you have already taken Prozac or one of its successors and know how it worked. Some of you would never think of a drug to help your anxiety, depression, or anger for fear it might do harm. Why read this third edition to discover whether the latest—Lexapro or Cymbalta—are worth trying? Are these two the miracle antidepressants their predecessors were not? The answer is, they are just as good but no better.

Then why this third edition (in only seven years)? The reason is that after having treated hundreds of people with these agents, read much of the available scientific literature on the subject, and spoken to as many specialists in the field as possible, it remains evident that these drugs are unable to cure about 30 to 40 percent of the people who take them. Here I will suggest new ways to help those who have previously not gotten better. In addition, as I will make clear in the first chapter, the controversies surrounding psychiatric medications influence prescribers and patients in ways that do much unseen harm.

Although it would be helpful to rename these drugs because

they are not just antidepressants, convention makes this impossible. Nonetheless, doctors and patients employ them for scores of other conditions, especially anxiety, for which they were not originally intended. By now, the "antidepressants" have been used for just about every psychiatric problem. It would be easier to construct a list of disorders for which they have not been used than the other way around.

Further experience with patients, reading of the literature, and talking with colleagues has also convinced me of the need to make explicit what many of the most thoughtful doctors and researchers confess in the halls after lectures. That is that the actions of these drugs on the neurotransmitters, serotonin, norepinephrine, and perhaps dopamine may have little or nothing to do with how they help you. It seems peculiar to me to construct a whole biochemical and neurological theory to try to explain agents that by and large help people only slightly more than a placebo does. The psychopharmacology historian David Healy describes in his excellent book, *The Creation of Psychopharmacology*, that Nathan Kline, the discoverer of one of the first antidepressants, Nardil, in 1957 warned against reliance on changes in rating scales as evidence of antidepressant treatment effect. Healy instead recommends "straightforward clinical observation . . . (to) show what a treatment is doing to help." Because penicillin is so powerful in its action, a controlled trial has never been necessary to prove its value. Similarly, Jean Delay, one of the discoverers in 1952 of Thorazine, the first antipsychotic, chided his American colleagues that with all their reverence for statistics, by the tenth patient it was clear that this drug provided a major breakthrough in the treatment of schizophrenia.

Symptoms or Syndrome?

Up until 1980, an individual was diagnosed as depressed solely because of depressed mood. Since 1980, the year the *Diagnostic and Statistical Manual of Mental Disorders*, Third Edition (*DSM* III) was published, this single symptom has been replaced by five of a list of nine symptoms, including a mood change, plus bodily alterations in sleep and appetite to diagnose the syndrome (a group of symptoms that collectively characterize a disease or disorder) major depressive disorder (MDD), which includes insomnia, fatigue, headache, and various bodily aches and pains. Someone suffering MDD may be irritable and anxious, while not feeling depressed at all.

Why the switch to a syndrome instead of just depressed mood? According to Philip G. Janicak et al., *Principles and Practice of Psychopharmacotherapy* (Williams and Wilkins), "Factor analysis of characteristics that distinguished drug versus placebo responders in clinical trials conducted in the early 1960s, when depressed mood was the single criterion for entry" showed a high placebo response rate and no difference could be shown in controlled drug versus placebo trials that the antidepressant was superior. It was only when the MDD syndrome, which included neurovegetative signs and symptoms, was constructed that the antidepressant could be shown to be statistically superior to placebo.

What Janicak et al. failed to make explicit in their text was that the syndrome MDD was styled by statisticians assembling this conglomerate in order to prove in a controlled and thus allegedly scientific way that these drugs were more effective than tonics or sugar pills. In spite of the claims of the framers of the *DSM* III, there is nothing more scientifically noteworthy about the diagnosis MDD than there was about the *DSM* II (1968) diagnosis of depression alone. Furthermore, the MDD syndrome, because of its listing requirement of five out of nine assembled a group of so-called depressives whose symptoms could make them very unlike one another. In addition, the syndrome creates a situation in which so-called antidepressants could settle the stomach, improve sleep, and thereby register as better by the Hamilton Depression Rating (HDR) scale, which has since been used in every controlled medication trial in order to scientifically prove drug superiority to placebo, a requirement necessary before the new drug would be approved by the Food and Drug Administration (FDA) for release to the public. MDD was a new illness invented by psychiatrists and the statisticians working under their supervision. Once the illness MDD had been created, the drug/placebo difference could then be established, and psychiatry could announce itself to be scientific and based on evidence. The statisticians had divided the many symptoms a *DSM* II depressed mood patient suffered (e.g., headaches, insomnia, sadness, pain, lack of appetite, loss of energy, diminished sexual drive, loss of motivation and interest, absence of pleasure, and low self-esteem). They found a cluster of these symptoms which, when grouped, could be shown to provide a drug/placebo difference. This became the foundation for the *DSM* III MDD, a new syndrome. A new illness had been invented to fit the pills designed to treat it.

Much of the same slight-of-hand trick has been charged by some critics of cognitive behavior therapy (CBT), the only psychotherapy that has presumed objective scientific backing in the treatment of depression. To prove its effectiveness scientifically, depression was redefined as due to various negative thoughts, which changed when the scale designed to show positive thoughts replacing the so-called depressed ones indicated it. Whether the pre-1980 (the year the American Psychiatric Association's revolutionary *DSM* III was published) *DSM* II (1968) depressed mood would have been changed significantly by CBT over its placebo was never tested.

What Happens After an Antidepressant Is Sanctioned by the FDA and Released?

All these careful diagnostic points defining MDD get lost in the typical busy doctor's office, and people who say they are depressed or anxious get the drug, and most of them feel better. By most, I mean about 60 percent, which closely resembles what would happen had they received a placebo, or

St. John's Wort, or an omega-3 fatty acid, or perhaps even a kind, supportive therapist willing to talk to them weekly. The latter is time-consuming and expensive. The primary care physician has no time, financial incentive, or interest in talk therapy.

But what is almost as interesting is what happens to the rest who recover only partially or not at all from antidepressant drug therapy. About 20 percent cannot tolerate it because of side effects such as abdominal distress, insomnia, a "drugged" feeling, or sexual difficulties. And another 20 percent get a little better, but not much. It is these two groups that provide the market for the latest and newest antidepressants.

What Are the FDA Rules Prior to Release?

The FDA requires two controlled double-blind randomized studies in which drug exceeds placebo on carefully selected (usually volunteers) "pure" MDD subjects, who are unlike people who are usually seen in clinical offices. These research subjects do not use alcohol or other drugs of abuse prior to entering the trial, and are not medically ill. Patients with all kinds of other reasons to be depressed, such as cancer, arthritis, heart or lung disease, anemia, job loss, poverty, physical or psychological abuse, death of a loved one, a recent divorce, other psychiatric conditions, are also excluded from these scientific drug trials. This is necessary because the drugs do not work in the presence of powerful depressing forces in a person's life, and because a pure sample of depressed patients must be assembled that is not contaminated by other illness in order to study the effect of an antidepressant on depression.

Despite all this careful selection, a remarkable problem has arisen in the research on all the new antidepressants. Most of them fail to surpass placebo. One author found that of forty carefully designed controlled studies of the five most commonly used specific serotonin reuptake inhibitors (SSRIs), only eight exceeded placebo. But the thirty-two failures were not revealed because the drug companies who sponsor the research at great cost are not required to publish the failures. If only your favorite baseball or football team could enjoy such gentle treatment: only have its victories recorded and not its defeats.

The Problem of Severity

Finally, there is the problem of the severity of the depression. Predictably, mild to moderate depression responds the best and severe depression the worst. But when one uses a drug placebo scientific and statistical model, the idea of response becomes tricky. Over 50 percent of mild depressions respond to drugs *and* to placebo. Almost all of the studies of the new antidepressants have been conducted on nonhospitalized, volunteer outpatients. The reason why it has been so difficult to show drug/placebo difference is that the placebo improvement rate is too high in many of those examined. Half of the drug and the placebo groups both get better. When severely depressed hospitalized people are looked at for four to six weeks (the conventional brief length of a study because they are so expensive to conduct), about 10 percent at best get better on placebo and 20 to 30 percent from a drug. Put another way, 70 percent or more remain severely ill, and may continue to be so for six months to a year. The few longer studies show the percentage of recoveries rising as the months pass. But the drug/placebo difference, curiously, is greater in the severely ill, although the overall recovery rate, that which ultimately truly counts for the patient (and the doctor) is low. In fact, unfortunately, about 20 percent of severe depressives never recover at all.

Why Not Just Give a Placebo to Mildly to Moderately Depressed Outpatients?

Placebos aren't given to mildly to moderately depressed outpatients because if the doctor told the patient the treatment consisted of an inert white powder, the person would be outraged, uncooperative, and the treatment would not work, nor would the individual be likely to see that physician again. And announcing it to be an active agent when it is not would be a lie. Curiously, the placebo was discovered on the battlefields of Italy during World War II. Harry Beecher, an anesthetist, had run out of morphine to calm the writhing wounded while the surgeon operated, and an enterprising nurse substituted saline (water and salt) intravenously and the wounded held still so the surgeon could proceed safely. The physician noted the miraculous effect on pain, and spent the rest of his life at Harvard, with a group he assembled, studying and teaching about the placebo. In my view, depression is psychic pain, often accompanied by physical pain, in the back, abdomen, or head. It should come as no surprise that the placebo works well in both depression and pain.

The Antidepressants Are, Nonetheless, Effective

Despite the shaky nature of the science behind the statistically made up syndrome of MDD, I have witnessed many occasions when these drugs have produced truly remarkable and lasting effects. I have a theory about why this is so that goes beyond the simple placebo. The medications are working in a way the laboratory scientists and drug company experimenters have failed to measure. Either they are causing people to sleep better, and thus to be less fatigued and depressed, or they are calming their upset stomachs and relieving their headaches.

Recently, almost all the new antidepressants have been approved as antianxiety agents, too. Cymbalta, the newest, is being cited for its pain relief. The old antidepressant Elavil (amitriptyline, 1961) also relieved pain, as do other antidepressants. Thus, they are calming people in a way the scientific scales do not capture. In fact, the standard HDR is composed of 40 percent anxiety items. In addition, they are making some people less irritable and thus easier to work and live with. Psychiatry currently has no name for disorders of anger, as it does for anxiety and depression. Nonetheless, anger is widely recognized by clinicians, relatives, and co-workers who come in contact with those who are irritable or enraged. But the *DSM* IV recognizes no formal diagnostic category of anger disorders, and thus it remains unstudied and largely ignored. As you might imagine, there is a proposal that anger disorders be included in the *DSM* V, scheduled for publication in 2007, recently postponed to 2012.

Treatment-Resistant Depression

This is the name given to those who do not recover from two separate four-to-six-week trials of the currently available antidepressants. They are then subjected to various unproven protocols in which other drugs are substituted or added, in the hope something will work. I will speak of these schemes in more detail later.

Would Treatment Resistance Be More Responsive If Psychiatrists Stopped Thinking About Major Depression as a Syndrome?

I believe the answer is yes, and I have found a small group of experts who have recommended specific symptoms be treated when the antidepressants fail. This approach requires people to reappraise why they are depressed, and to carefully review what they mean, not what the experts mean, when they say they are depressed. It encourages people to really think about what is making them feel badly and what symptoms brought them to their physician in the first place.

The Causes of Depression

Depression has as many causes as do pain and fever. It extends from an unhappy marriage to an unbearable job; a narrow, boring life; the abuse of a nasty or controlling boss or family; an undetected or chronic physical illness; a traumatic experience; a feeling of spiritual emptiness; a lack of hope that tomorrow will be better; loneliness; or whatever else a person discovers when taking a personal inventory. It may be useful to review these causes with a therapist, one with an open mind who tries to help you discover the cause within yourself, rather than one who has a theory, whether it be of abuse, or of bad mothers, or negative thoughts, or lack of religion, or a need for a baby, or for recognition, or a bad diet, or a brain allergy. Watch out for cranks who either say nothing at all or try to persuade you that they, rather than you, have the answer to your depression. I have also noticed a few people who, try as they might, are unable to come up with a reason for why they feel badly. The psychoanalyst would blame the unconscious and the biological psychiatrist would attribute the disorder to bad genes or a chemical imbalance. These represent their theories and not established, scientific fact. The unconscious does not, after years of psychoanalysis, reveal the cause of depression, and thus make it go away, and no one has ever proven that a chemical imbalance or a gene for depression exists. Some people (the minority) are depressed, and no one can discover why.

What Is the Symptom for Which You Need Help?

This is where some psychiatrists, especially when encountering people who do not respond to antidepressants, are beginning to go back to the pre-1960 symptom treatment approach. If you cannot sleep and this robs your life of pleasure and energy, take a sleeping pill. They work better than antidepressants for insomnia. If fear is robbing your life of pleasure, take an antianxiety benzodiazepine such as Valium or Klonopin to calm it, if all other measures have failed, and do not worry about addiction to it. In many ways, the old antianxiety agents, the Ativans and the Xanaxes, act more quickly, with fewer side effects, and are the most commonly used drugs in medical offices to this day, although this fact is hidden by the glossy, color ads in medical journals, in popular magazines, and on TV, because the antianxiety agents are all generic, since the patents have expired, and the drug companies have no financial incentive to promote them. They would rather offer Effexor XR or other SSRIs, still under patent protection, for millions of dollars in revenue, although practically no one (I have seen occasional exceptions) has matched them up against the benzodiazepines (the Valiums, Klonopins, Xanaxes, and Ativans), probably for fear that not only are the new antidepressants not better for anxiety, but they require one to three weeks to take effect; they cause upset stomach; insomnia, impotence, and other sexual dysfunctions; and no one has ever proven that they are less addictive. They are simply newer, more costly, and if someone tries to stop taking Effexor XR suddenly instead of gradually and carefully, they will suffer just as they would if they suddenly discontinued a benzodiazepine. Needless to say, no one has put my last statement to the comparative test, because there is no financial incentive to do so, and not enough noncorporate funds available to do all the research needed.

If you lack energy and barely can drag yourself out of bed, and collapse back on the couch after work, and there is no medical reason for it, you might be better off not thinking you have a treatment-resistant depression, but that you need a stimulant, such as Provigil, a new drug which is frequently effective.

I will not add each possible symptom and its treatment in this section. After all, it is meant to be an introduction, not the book itself. This new edition will list all the symptomatic treatments available, instead of confining itself to the "scientifically established" syndromes and their antidepressant drug treatment that my previous two did. I feel I have finally broken loose from serotonin and norepinephrine and from the statisticians' artificially constructed MDD syndrome. But it still remains useful to think about which symptoms might naturally occur together. For example, Rosalind D. Cartwright has suggested research on the relationship between sleep disturbance and daily moods. Does the depression cause the insomnia or does the insomnia cause the depression? This question is not an example of academic nit-picking, but has the practical implication of whether to treat with an antidepressant or a hypnotic. Of course, in the busy world of clinical medicine, the patient is likely to get both drugs, that is, if the physician is not opposed to sleeping pills because of fear patients will become addicted.

Whose Advice Should I Follow About Whether or Not to Take a Psychiatric Drug?

Beliefs influence all medical decisions, but their power is greatest on psychiatric treatments. Some people are reluctant to take medicine for any illness, while others run to the pill cabinet and cannot wait to try the latest. Emotion not only governs drug taking, but whether one goes to doctors at all, seeks out or avoids a surgeon even for emergency procedures, not just optional ones. As in most beliefs, there are those of which we are fully aware and others that affect us without our realizing.

Beliefs: Their Influence on Medical Decisions

Neither you nor I have ever heard a debate about whether a person should take digitalis for heart disease. There simply is no controversy regarding this decision. Some medical judgments do arouse considerable disagreement, such as stomach stapling for obesity, narcotics for chronic pain, plastic surgery to undo the signs of aging, the "morning-after" pill for unprotected intercourse, the need for and frequency of periodic checkups of the whole body or various individual parts of it, such as the eyes, the skin, the colon, the breasts, the prostate, and the teeth. One's beliefs and fears powerfully influence doctor-seeking and doctor-avoiding behavior. Some ignore the whole matter, adopting the fatalistic view that when one's number is up, it's up. Others seek solace in nonmedical settings, go to a house of worship, a shaman, an acupuncturist, the gym, or alter their diet (if you eat natural foods, you'll live longer), or try to cultivate optimism in the belief it will add years to their lives. A few move away from what they view as toxic cities in order to live in sections of the world noted for longevity.

The Treatment of Anxiety, Depression, and Other Psychiatric Disorders

If there were a shortage of doctors and a plague occurred, medicine would concern itself only with life-and-death matters, and ignore obesity, face-lifts, and tooth whitening. If psychiatrists were confronted with the completely insane and violent, feeling nervous or unhappy would similarly become unimportant. A psychiatric disorder is defined in the context of the society and the resources available to combat it.

There is no doubt that a psychiatric plague exists in our modern era. Junior high school students murder their classmates, teachers, and families. Addicts commit violent crimes to get money for their habits. Anorexics starve to death. Suicide continues and perhaps increases among the young. Severe mental illness remains uncured, its victims homeless in our streets and occupying our jails, as we continue to close our mental facilities, not fund treatment, and fail to pay for fundamental research necessary to provide answers to this lingering horror. We fire one thousand cruise missiles at a cost of $600,000 each, while ignoring the suffering of those within our borders.

Mild to Moderate Depression, Anxiety, and Anger

While necessity requires us to allocate scarce public funds to the most severely ill, mild to moderate depression and anxiety ought not to be ignored, even if it must be paid for by private insurance or out of pocket. These mild to moderate mood disorders take a terrible toll on the modern family and the workplace. Epidemiologists have revealed the costs in dollars and in surprisingly enormous psychological harm to marriage, children, workers, the gross national product, and the future of our nation. Although the symptom picture may be greeted with scorn by mental health workers taking care of chronic, impaired schizophrenics, the violently insane, the severe addicts, criminals, and murderers, it has been shown time and time again by careful researchers that mild to moderate mood disorders deserve our attention.

I will only give a few examples here of the hundreds that could be included regarding the damage caused by so-called mild to moderate mood disorders. Seventy percent of doctors' visits are devoted to such patients, who often require expensive laboratory tests, all of which add to the already overburdened medical costs we face both as individuals and within our corporations, which have to compete with those in the rest of the world, where such niceties go unnoticed. An irritable mother or father can harm a child's growth and development on a daily basis, doing more cumulative damage than that caused by more dramatic one-time occurrences, such as divorce, job loss, illness, or poverty. A continuously depressed parent, unable to feed, care for, discipline, or teach a child harms the next generation, even though the mental disorder would be termed mild or moderate by the classifiers. A chronically anxious, worried, depressed parent undermines the confidence of their offspring, strains the marriage, and is a poor economic provider, because their mood disorder detracts from their work performance. Self-medication with alcohol or drugs by people suffering mild to moderate mood disorders does enormous damage, with little fanfare or notice. Drunk drivers on our roads kill ten times as many each year as we lost in the World Trade Center disaster. The cost of alcoholism on work and family is huge, and a large part of the drinking done is in the attempt to relieve the suffering caused by the so-called mild to moderate mood disorders. Several British authors have referred contemptuously to such people as "the nervous populace," but I take strong exception to such dismissal of their suffering and its effects.

How Does Your Belief System Perceive a Mild to Moderate Mood Disorder?

Obviously, this depends on your temperament, religious conviction, and life view. You can ignore and deny the whole matter, interpret it as a physical condition, view it as weak and shameful, self-medicate it with drugs and alcohol, consider it retribution from God for your sins, blame it on others (your meaningless job, your unloving family, your abusive spouse, your critical mother or cold father, your diet, your genes, or your chemistry). I will not attempt to list all the possibilities: the physical ones (undetected medical illnesses), the spiritual ones (a poor relationship with God, the earth, a lack of real values), physical or psychological abuse, no exercise, the failure to connect meaningfully with others, a useless job, an unfulfilling marriage, pessimism about the future, or the lack of strength to face aging and, eventually, death.

How Do You Feel About Psychiatric Treatment in General?

This runs the gamut from totally unnecessary, a sign of weakness, that it is ineffective and useless, to one regarding it as enlightened and the only hope. Within the category of psychiatric treatments, which could be compared to the general belief in God, are the various religions: drugs, psychoanalysis, psychodynamic psychotherapy, supportive psychotherapy, CBT, interpersonal psychotherapy, and the approximately one hundred other psychotherapies. Each of these religions has its liberal members willing to try one or more houses of worship in their search for help, and their rigid devotees committed only to one of them. Since this book is devoted to the drug treatment of mild to moderate mood disorders, and is not a general psychiatric text, I will devote the rest of this introduction to the conscious and unconscious attitudes people have toward drugs designed to relieve anxiety, depression, insomnia, and irritability. Naturally, the unconscious ones are more interesting.

How This Third Edition Completely Differs from the First Two

The first two editions portrayed the excitement of treating depression with brand-new safe and effective agents. As time has passed, Prozac, Paxil, and several other antidepressants have been released in generic form. Not only are they no longer new, they have been better studied and understood. Many of them have received official FDA recognition for the treatment of generalized anxiety disorder, panic disorder, social anxiety disorder, obsessive-compulsive disorder, and posttraumatic stress disorder. Thus, they have a prominent role in the treatment of the anxiety disorders. This is responsible for the beginning in the change in focus of this edition.

Thus, liberated in my thinking because of the inclusion of anxiety, I began to wonder about the other major mood disorder, although it is not officially recognized in the *DSM* IV. This is the disorder of anger, which is being considered as an addition for *DSM* V, and is either ignored or scattered within *DSM* IV, so as to be almost invisible. As I reviewed the second edition of my book, I noticed that the anger disorder is included, but only in passing references, rather than being awarded equal status. This third edition corrects the imbalance in the previous two.

The Role of (Conscious and Unconscious) Beliefs and Attitudes in the Drug Treatment of Mild to Moderate Mood Disorders

1. I Would Never Take a Drug for a Mood Disorder.

The reasons for this vary extensively from person to person. For some, it means admitting one is sick and weak. For others, it implies losing control over one's own moods and turning their management over to a drug.

2. I Would Prefer to Take a Drug.

To many people, influenced by the conversion of psychiatry from psychoanalysis to biology, biochemistry, and genetics, mood disorders are conceived of as chemical imbalances, much like diabetes, and should be treated by a drug in order to restore body chemistry. Thus, the condition is not the sufferer's fault, just as diabetes is not, and people need not blame themselves for being unable to control their emotions. The former stigma of mental illness is thus avoided by the ethical and moral exemption one is granted because one is sick.

3. Taking a Drug Means I Am Sicker Than If I Only Participate in Psychotherapy.

Psychiatric residents queried at Columbia Medical School were much happier admitting to being in psychoanalysis than taking medications for mood disorders. If professional psychiatrists in advanced training feel this way about drugs, it is no wonder that a significant portion of the general population does, too.

4. The Doctor's or Therapist's Attitude.

When someone does not feel well, as they usually do not when suffering from a mood disorder, they look to their psychiatrist, family physician, or psychotherapist for guidance. If the care provider is antidrug, they feel worse when they need or want to be medicated, or they may refuse drugs because of the advice of or contempt they sense from their therapist. Thus, they may remain in pain longer than necessary. If the treater believes drugs cover up and paper over problems, then the therapist regards their use as failures of his or her own skills or questions the resolve of the patient to grow and conquer problems.

5. The Negative Press Received by the SSRIs.

In general, medical drugs do not give rise to the levels of screaming controversy among doctors themselves, or other interested people, which makes rational discourse about them difficult. Prozac, for example, has been accused of being a stimulant, addictive, of causing violence and suicide, of inducing impulsive and grandiose behaviors, of producing tics and abnormal movements, of worsening depression, of causing permanent brain dysfunction and damage to the serotonin system, and of inducing madness. It has been charged with interfering with memory and motor performance. The Federal Aviation Administration, for example, does not allow pilots to take Prozac. I believe this is a mistake, since I would rather have a nondepressed pilot who is on Prozac, a drug that does not interfere with motor skills, than a depressed one who is considering death.

Then there are the opposing views that Prozac not only is safe, but restores lives, cures depression, and has provided a significant contribution to the alleviation of suffering. What to make of the bad reports about the antidepressants? The answer, say advocates of drug use, is that 25 million people have taken them, and of these some have committed murder or suicide, or have severe brain disorders, are psychotic, or have neurological disease. Is it the drug's fault, or random occurrence in such a huge population? Can anything be made of it at all? All medical treatments have helped (one hopes) more people than they have harmed or killed. It must be remembered that some cures and calamities occur separately from the drug altogether. Why do critics like Dr. Peter Breggin attribute such power to Prozac to do evil on the one hand, while at the same time accusing it of being little more than a placebo? It seems to me such experts have an axe to grind. These pro- and antidrug camps seem to be more like the radical right and left screaming at each other on the Chris Matthews show on MSNBC, than like sober scientists.

6. The Special Case of the Benzodiazepines.

Once they were relegated to the world of anxiety, and since depression was the focus, they were neglected (including by me in the first two editions of this book). Now that anxiety disorders have achieved equal status with depression (and anger disorders are creeping into focus), the role of the benzodiazepines is again being noticed. A further reason for their having been ignored is that they have been around for almost fifty years, are all generic, and make no money for the major drug companies. The academic doctors, many of whom are supported personally in some cases by amounts up to $1,000,000 per year, while also having their research funded, seemed happy to ignore the old benzodiazepines (the Valiums, Ativans, Xanaxes, and Klonopins) in favor of the rich antidepressants.

Now the antidepressants are slowly joining the antianxiety agents (benzodiazepines) in the drug historical warehouse. Meantime, the benzodiazepines have not been forgotten. Even at the peak of Prozac excitement, they have been used by doctors across America twice as often as antidepressants. But they suffer from the stigma of being addicting and thus dangerous, the same charge that Dr. Peter Breggin (*Talking Back to Prozac*) has brought against Prozac.

The antianxiety agents frequently double as hypnotic agents to treat insomnia. They are carefully delineated in the *PDR* (*Physician's Desk Reference*) by the drug companies as only working for three weeks, unless this limit is overruled by a doctor. Although people have successfully taken them for twenty-five years or more without becoming addicted, escalating the dose, losing the effect, or frying their brains, the drug companies want to transfer any legal liabilities occurring after three weeks to the prescribing doctor. I will speak more of this in the new section on the benzodiazepines, which I essentially overlooked in the first two editions.

Getting Help

If you decide that you have a clinical depression in need of treatment, the first thing you need to do is get professional help. Since this is a book on antidepressant medication, I will concentrate on these agents, but for most depressed patients, psychotherapy is equally important. While my discussion of psychotherapy will be necessarily brief, it is essential that anyone seeking treatment for depression have a good idea of what help to expect from drugs and what issues require talk therapy, for it is in the combination of the two that the best hope lies.

The first step in getting help is to find a good therapist. Physicians, clergy, friends, and relatives can be excellent sources for a recommendation. If none of these are available, try the local medical or psychiatric society or a nearby medical school. Consider your first visit a trial in which you evaluate what is said to you and whether you feel comfortable with the person you see. It is essential not only that you like the therapist, but that they impress you with their capacity to understand your situation and have something helpful to tell you. If the therapist is not a physician and you require an antidepressant, then either your own doctor or a psychiatrist will have to prescribe it. Once this is done, the therapist and the doctor who prescribed the medication must confer regularly about your progress. If you are already in psychotherapy with a nonphysician and also wish to try an antidepressant, discuss it with your therapist. Most will welcome the possibility of adding medication to ease your pain, but a minority may accuse you of dodging responsibility and seeking an easy way out. This minority does not understand that psychotherapy and antidepressants work better together for depressed people than either does alone.

The chapters that follow discuss the mood disorders (depression, anxiety, and anger), how they are treated, and describe the groups of drugs that are being widely used to combat them. It is my hope that this book will help you find the answers you are looking for and start you on the road to a happier, healthier life.

THE NEW ANTIDEPRESSANTS

AND

ANTIANXIETIES

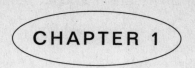

CHAPTER 1

Understanding Mood Disorders (Depression, Anxiety, and Anger)

Before discussing treatment in detail, it is important to understand exactly what these mood disorders are and how they are diagnosed. This chapter takes you step-by-step through their symptoms and diagnosis.

The Symptoms of a Major Depressive Episode

Although the term *clinical depression* is commonly used, the precise term is *major depression*, which is what I will use throughout this book. The symptoms of major depression are the following:

Depressed Mood

A depressed mood is a constant sad, dejected feeling lasting at least two weeks, which must be differentiated from normal blues or discouragement. Although the difference between feeling sad and depression can be hard to distinguish in words, those who have experienced both have little difficulty in telling them apart.

Hopelessness is central to this mood, a feeling that there is nothing to look forward to and that the pain will never cease. This desperate, miserable feeling can be accompanied by excessive worry about anything or everything, including money, health, family, work, and friendships.

A depressed mood can be the most painful affliction a human can suffer. Depressed patients who break a leg or get pneumonia welcome the physical pain as a distraction from their extreme psychological discomfort. Their gloomy pessimism allows them no hope of escape from their agony. They do not expect to get well.

Depressed people may find themselves bursting into tears without warning. They may run from the sight of others, embarrassed by their loss of control.

Being in a depressed mood can make one excessively sensitive and "thin-skinned," quick to take offense, easily hurt and discouraged. The depressed person can overreact to his own errors and therefore be unwilling to take chances and try new or difficult tasks. At work, depressives are timid, afraid to be inventive, and most comfortable with routine assignments.

Depressives can be irritable, and some are subject to sudden rages. They are often short on patience and bristle for little or no reason.

The mood of the depressive may or may not be influenced by actual events. Some are highly reactive, instantly lifted by praise or thrown to the depths by criticism. Such individuals are viewed by friends and colleagues as requiring very careful handling. People walk on eggshells around them. The insensitive spouse has no recognition of how much he influences his depressive partner's mood. One thoughtless boss's praise and criticism caused his depressed assistant to go from joy to gloom because of her exquisite sensitivity. Other depressives show little reaction to the good things that happen to them. In fact, they seem only to register the bad, particularly the slights and criticisms they encounter. Some experts have judged the unreactive depressives to be more severe, but it may be that they are just different. If a patient were to commit suicide in reaction to rejection, to call such a depression less severe makes no sense.

The pain of the depressed mood makes the sufferer seek relief in a large variety of actions, ranging from harmless to life-threatening. The unhappy go shopping, take a vacation, change jobs, careers, even spouses, while the acutely tormented drink too much, take drugs, or induce pain by relentlessly picking at their fingers or cutting themselves in an attempt to relieve the pain in their head.

A depressed mood often influences the way a depressive relates to others. Some seek out friends and loved ones in an effort to feel better by being with people. The pain of their illness makes them more dependent on others. They call their friends and relatives incessantly on the phone, require their spouse to listen to them endlessly, and wear everyone out with inordinate demands on their time. Often their complaints and concerns are dull and repetitious. Some seem to ask for advice, which they then ignore, frustrating those giving it. Such people feel much worse when alone. Others seek solitude and find being with people a strain—false and meaningless. They hide when depressed, call no one, do not answer their phone, and, when forced to communicate with others, do so monosyllabically.

Loss of Interest or Pleasure in Activities

When loss of interest or pleasure in activities is sudden and all-inclusive, it is easy for the patient, the family, and the doctor to recognize. For example, a previously lively and involved working mother stops caring about her job or children, and only wants to stay in bed and do nothing. She is clearly experiencing a decline of interest and pleasure in her usual activities. When the change is more gradual and selective in its targets, it can be more difficult to evaluate. For example, the loss of satisfaction may initially be limited to responsibilities and obligations, while the desire for recreational activities and vacations increases. A woman may say she hates her job or even her husband, but will continue to enjoy long lunches or trips to Europe. A student may stop studying or going to class, but will spend time skiing and partying. The person who says that being a lawyer or shopkeeper is no longer interesting is often depressed rather than merely ready for a career change. When a man says he no longer loves his wife of seventeen years, he may hide the underlying depressive cause of his loss of pleasure in her company in seemingly normal-sounding phrases, such as "we have grown apart," "she is immature," "she only cares about clothes and appearances." Many depressions are missed by the patient, the family, and even the doctor because they are described in terms that seem understandable and not pathological. Before you change your job or spouse, find out whether your misery is due to a major depression rather than circumstances outside you. The distinction between internally and externally caused depression can be difficult and may require the help of a psychiatrist.

The loss of interest and pleasure affects one's ability to plan for the future, especially long-term. This absence of spontaneous motivation means the sufferer will do only that which he or she is forced to do, either by necessity or by an employer. This condition has been described as a paralysis of will, in which the point of doing anything at all seems lost. Goals that once attracted—the desire for money, fame, prestige, success—no longer seem worthwhile. The notion that "there is no point" and that "life is futile" takes over in the absence of pleasure.

In the deepest depressions, when all interest and pleasure is gone, the sufferer has no desire to do anything. There is no gratification from food or sex. Psychiatrists take the inability to work and the cessation of all sexual desire as signs of the deepest depression, requiring prompt and rigorous treatment.

Can You Be Depressed Without a Depressed Mood?

To be diagnosed as having a depression you must be suffering from *either* a depressed mood *or* a loss of interest and pleasure in usual activities, but not necessarily both. How can someone be depressed without a depressed mood? Sometimes it is because the person does not recognize the mood or will not admit to it. Those who consider depression to have the stigma of mental illness fight the recognition. Others consider long periods of low mood to be a normal part of life for which there is no diagnosis or treatment. Some patients do not complain of sadness but appear depressed, and occasionally will admit it when others point it out. Major depressives may suffer severe aches and pains in the stomach, back, or head, but do not say they feel unhappy. These bodily equivalents of the mental pain associated with a depressed mood often respond to antidepressant drug therapies. Patients with major depressive disorder can suffer from other aspects of the illness but not from a depressed mood. They may tell their friends, family, even their doctors that they cannot sleep, have severe headaches or stomachaches, that they are exhausted, but not that they have a depressed mood. It is up to the doctor to recognize and treat such people for depression. Unfortunately, the diagnosis is often missed. One study found that over 70 percent of such patients were not diagnosed by their medical doctors as depressed when they should have been, and thus they underwent many unnecessary tests for physical illness and failed to be relieved of their depression.

Bodily Changes

Changes in weight, sleep patterns, activity, and energy levels are characteristic of major depression.

Weight

Although weight and appetite may be significantly increased or decreased, the most typical pattern is that of weight loss accompanied by little desire for food. The depressed patient may lose 5 percent of his or her body weight within a month without dieting. This can be alarming and may trigger a medical workup to make sure an organic illness is not the cause. Less severely depressed patients may eat too much. Some say food is comforting and makes them feel better, while others have cravings for sweets and other high-caloric foods. One such woman gained fifty pounds in one year.

Sleep

The most typical major depressive sleep disturbance involves awakening in the middle of the night and finding it very difficult or impossible to go back to sleep. The patient's day may begin at three or four in the morning, making him or her appear and feel exhausted. In addition, the depressive may also have trouble falling asleep. A minority of depressives sleep too much, finding their only pleasure in escaping from the world. One woman would do only what she had to do for the care of her family and otherwise spent most of her life in bed. She could think of nothing more enjoyable to do with her time. But most depressives complain constantly of their inability to sleep. They dread getting into bed and facing another long sleepless night. They beg for sleeping pills to help them rest.

Activity

There are two types of activity changes occurring in major depressives: agitation and retardation. Agitation is a state of constant restless motion which in major depressives can take the form of pacing aimlessly, hand-wringing, and being unable to sit still. For purposes of formal diagnosis, the condition must be severe enough so that the agitation is noticeable to others. Retardation, also objectively observable, is evident in movement and in speech. There is a slowing of thought and verbal response. The patient has almost nothing to say spontaneously and answers questions monosyllabically or not at all. Such a person is boring to be with and hard to talk to.

Energy

A depressed person with low energy may awaken tired or become easily wearied by normal physical or mental effort. Even previously simple tasks seem a burden. Letters remain unanswered, even unopened, while routine tasks take longer. Anything new or out of the ordinary is avoided. This loss of energy may be wrongly attributed to physical illness, and a series of expensive medical tests may be ordered. Or the patient may conclude that overwork is responsible and go on vacation, which provides temporary relief, but no permanent solution. Chronic fatigue syndrome can sometimes be due to unrecognized depression.

The seeming laziness of the depressed patient who appears unwilling to perform energetically either at work or at home can make employers and family extremely angry. If there were a physical cause, like pneumonia, others would be more forgiving. But depression is not a physical illness and the patient's loss of spontaneous motivation and movement can frustrate those around him because they do not understand the illness.

Thinking Changes

Thoughts of worthlessness or guilt, a diminished ability to think or concentrate, indecisiveness, and recurrent thoughts of death or suicide are also characteristics of major depression.

Sense of Worthlessness or Guilt

The overwhelming majority of depressed patients do not like themselves, denouncing themselves as inadequate in terms of all the qualities that they value: attractiveness, intelligence, and popularity. They feel ugly, stupid, unlovable, boring, and expect failure and rejection. They regard themselves as unequal to the tasks they attempt, and the more severely ill feel loathed by all who know them and deserving of severe punishment. No matter how successful they in fact are, they regard themselves as failures: millionaires feel poor, serious authors feel like hacks. But what of the average man and woman who say they have done nothing with their lives? Are they right? They fail to credit themselves with having taken care of their families, done careful, high-quality, and useful work, helped their communities and churches. Instead they see only what they have not done, castigating themselves as poor parents, bad citizens, and slipshod workers. They focus on failures, ignore successes, and are filled with self-reproaches and self-blame. Depending on the severity of the condition, the patient experiences anything from self-dislike to self-hatred. There is a great disparity between the person's self-image and objective fact.

Guilt overwhelms them: they believe they have done terrible things, caused others great harm, and should be punished. Excessively self-blaming, the depressed person feels responsible for anything that goes wrong. A mother whose son failed an exam in elementary school believed it was her fault for not making him study enough and in the right way. A man who could not earn enough money to indulge his family's most elaborate whim thought himself a failure rather than concluding that they spent too much. When committing a minor error, the depressed patient exaggerates both its magnitude and the terrible consequences it might produce. The depressed woman feels she deserves to suffer for her sins and is filled with self-reproaches and self-blame.

Diminished Ability to Think or Concentrate, or Indecisiveness

The depressed patient's capacity to think can be severely disturbed and seem like a demented person's inability to concentrate or remember. A student's grades may drop sharply and a worker's performance deteriorate completely. Indecisiveness can slow or totally disrupt a patient's ability to function. It is caused by an inability to concentrate and do the work of choosing among alternatives to pick a course of action, and by the expectation that things will not turn out well. In fact, indecisiveness is a by-product of several of the symptoms of depression: the inability to concentrate, the sense that one's efforts will never succeed, the tendency to become easily tired when attempting difficult tasks, the low self-esteem that makes the worker feel unequal to the task, and the slowing and poverty of thoughts and ideas. The depressed patient's IQ can test lower because of disturbance in concentration, failure in memory, fatigue, and loss of motivation. It is not just that the depressed patient feels unwell; it may indeed be that the brain works less well. But whether the ultimate cause is a disorder of mood or of thought or both, the damage to the person's performance is devastating.

Recurrent Thoughts of Death, Thoughts of or Attempts at Suicide

Severe depression can be a fatal disease in 5 to 15 percent of those who suffer from it. The pain of this illness makes thoughts of death or action to seek it seem a welcome relief. Many patients contemplating suicide keep their thoughts and plans to themselves. Those who speak of it openly should not be dismissed as mere attention-getters, but be taken seriously. Many suicide attempts fail not because the individual is merely seeking attention but because of poor planning at a time when the person is very upset. Friends and relatives must be aware of this danger and act to stop it. If you feel hopeless and are thinking of killing yourself to end your misery, you must understand that depression is a treatable disease and you can be helped.

Four Common Ways the Diagnosis of Major Depression and Other Mood Disorders Can Be Missed

The Pain Way

Donna is thirty-seven years old and living in a new city, having been transferred by her company. She works sixty hours a week and comes home to an empty apartment on a street of strangers. Her stomach has been bothering her for months now, and lately the pain keeps her up at night. She worries that she may have an ulcer or worse, and has made several appointments with her doctor, who, after prescribing antacids without success, has scheduled her for X rays to have a look at her stomach and intestines. The films have come back normal, and he recommends a psychiatric consultation. Donna agrees to go. Many people would not, offended that the doctor does not regard the pain as real. Donna worries that her medical doctor might think her crazy, but decides not to say anything about it. Her distress has made her willing to try anything.

Donna's psychiatric interview reveals a depressed mood, and feelings of sadness, loneliness, and boredom. These symptoms have occurred over the last several months as Donna was leaving her old job and starting her new one. She took little interest or pleasure in her daily life and forced herself through the workday, collapsing at home at the end. She has lost fifteen pounds in the last month and awakens in the middle of the night and finds herself unable to get back to sleep. Doing her job has become more and more of a chore. She finds it difficult to keep up with the mail or return phone calls and has little energy to go out on sales calls.

Donna, like many depressed people, experienced her main symptom in the form of pain. Some suffer headaches, others backaches, and many, like Donna, have abdominal disturbances. When busy medical doctors do not question these individuals for the other symptoms of depression, the diagnosis is often missed. Not all the fault of lack of proper treatment lies with hurried or careless doctors. Many patients are unwilling to go to a psychiatrist or to listen to their family physician's recommendations of treatment for depression. The stigma of mental illness prevents many sufferers from getting the help they need.

The Fatigue Way

Claire is fifty-two years old. Her children have left home and her job as a real estate agent has produced declining income for her. She wonders if it's the rising interest rates or increased competition, but she feels less inclined to work with the clients she has or to seek new ones. She finds her household chores more daunting and feels little inclination to cook for her husband when he comes home from work. She sits and watches TV and lies around in bed. Her energy is so low that she has gone to several doctors to find out if her thyroid activity is low or if she is anemic. She even fears she may have some hidden cancer. But after numerous tests, nothing can be found. She becomes very angry when a psychiatric consultation is finally recommended. Her mother had been a serious depressive and Claire knows she is nothing like her. Perhaps she has chronic fatigue syndrome, but the possible viral cause cannot in her case be proved.

Unfortunately, Claire adamantly refuses psychiatric help. She is terrified she may have a version of her mother's depression. In fact, she does. She takes little interest or pleasure in her daily life, feels hopeless about her prospects for getting better, no longer enjoys sex with her husband, and feels anger toward him for requiring meals and her attention. She has difficulty falling asleep and awakens for long periods; sometimes she is unable to go back to sleep at all. She looks tired and grim. Her thoughts have slowed and she makes little spontaneous conversation. It has been months since she could concentrate and read a book.

If you are fighting the recognition that you are depressed out of fear that you are crazy or morally defective, remember that depression is a painful illness for which there is effective treatment. You can be helped, but you must admit your need!

The Hate Way

John is a forty-one-year-old stockbroker who over the past year has come to hate his wife. He began to have affairs. Several times he thought he was in love with someone else, but each time would be drawn back home to try to make his marriage work, not only for the sake of the children but also because he believed in the preservation of the family. He did not like thinking of himself as just another midlife-crisis sufferer off chasing women. He would return and try, but he could not stand his wife. He thought her values superficial, that all she cared about was lunches with her friends and making social dates with other couples. He found her long rehashes of their socializing insufferable, and her desire to talk out their problems made him want to run away. He hated the way she made love to him, which he believed was motivated by her wish to hang on to him rather than by honest sexual desire. John pretended to participate in the couples therapies she would drag him to, but would find ways not to continue going.

The feeling "I no longer love my wife" is a common manifestation of major depression. John's depression makes him lose interest in, and derive no pleasure from, other people, including his wife, and the hatred caused by his mood disorder focuses on her. At the same time, his illness makes John very needy and he keeps returning to the wife he hates. The momentary antidepressant effect of his affairs cannot replace the comfort of his family. He hates his wife and he cannot leave her.

John does not cling to a physical causation, as do those in pain or suffering fatigue, but he does not know he has a depressive illness either. Because he is tortured by his wish for family connection and his hatred of his wife, he is less resistant to counseling. But the counselor may not realize that the underlying cause of his marital problems is not primarily communication difficulties or an immature lack of commitment or his having outgrown or grown apart from his wife, or his recent discovery after twenty years of marriage that she is an "airhead," but the illness of depression. While talking to the counselor about his feelings toward his wife and the importance of maintaining the family may relieve him somewhat and teach him communication skills that are truly useful, the depressive illness must be addressed or the patient and the marriage cannot recover.

John has many of the symptoms of major depressive disorder obscured by the dramatic one that he hates his wife. He suffers from depressed mood, loss of pleasure, sleep disturbance; he has lost weight, has little energy, and feels guilty. John's depression is destroying his family and urgently needs to be treated.

The Job Way

Jeff is a successful lawyer, and has been for twelve years. Married with two kids, he has worked hard for his partnership and house in suburban New York. He needs his large salary, but for the last year he has found the law boring. There seems no point in helping one large corporation get or keep money away from another. Finding the simple winning line in a complicated litigation no longer excites him. He would like to do something that has more social value, like teaching disadvantaged children or helping the sick. But the thought of a second career, especially a low-paying one, seems out of the question. What would happen to his home, and how would he pay the private school tuition?

Joe is an auto mechanic who no longer takes any pleasure in discovering what is wrong with a customer's car and fixing it. Several years ago he switched from a large garage to a much smaller one so that he would have more personal contact with the individual car owner. For a while this seemed to cheer him up, but lately he no longer cares, even when he is complimented on his excellent work. The challenge is gone; the work seems dirty and arduous; and he wishes he could go back to school and become an engineer who designs cars, rather than a grease monkey working on them. But the change seems impossible, and he drags himself along, dreaming on, from day to day.

The lawyer and the auto mechanic just described have been referred to as "burned out," "in midlife crisis," narcissistic, immature, needing to grow up and face adult responsibility, and requiring a spiritual awakening. In fact, these two men are depressed; their depressed mood is expressed in their boredom and hopelessness, their loss of interest and pleasure in their work (not their loved ones), their troubled sleep, their lessened energy, their diminished ability to concentrate, their slowed thoughts and movements on the job. But they do not go to a psychiatrist and say they are depressed. They do not see themselves as depressed, and do not recognize their change in mood, thinking, behavior, and physical capacity as depression. Their spouses, families, friends, physicians, and vocational counselors also do not realize they are ill.

Do You Have Depression, a Mood Disorder, or Is This Simply Life?

The abrupt onset of symptoms in each of the four categories of depression (mood, mind, behaviors, and body) makes the diagnosis fairly obvious, if not for the sufferer, then at least for the family, friends, or psychiatrist. When the mood is depressed, the mind disinterested, unable to concentrate, indecisive, filled with self-loathing and suicidal thoughts, when the behavior is constantly restless or completely slowed, when the body is altered by sleep disturbance, appetite or weight change, frequent pain, or loss of sexual interest, then the diagnosis is obvious. But when you are angry, bored, worried, or unhappy, and you think you know the cause (your job, your spouse, your ungrateful children, or whatever else you hold responsible for your hopeless misery), you ought to consider the possibility of major depressive or other mood disorder being responsible. When you get the right cause and effective treatment, you will be saved a lot of suffering, not to mention needless divorces and job changes.

A significant percentage of my patients remain uncertain about whether to start antidepressant or other medication. They explore the deep hurts and abuses of their early childhoods in psychotherapy, or just go out and live life without outside help. Some of them are open to my opinion on the choice of therapy; others are not. Most of you reading this book either are simply curious about antidepressant or other drugs or are considering taking one. By the time most people pick up a book like this or consult a psychiatrist, they have been in pain for a long time and are unable to get out of it on their own. It is, in my opinion, a sign of health to know when to ask for help. While self-sufficiency is admirable, knowing when to seek assistance is intelligent. Of course, the decision has to do not with logic but with emotion, and many people are opposed to sharing their pain with anyone, even a professional. Progress has been made in the public's acceptance of psychiatric illness, but there's a long way to go, and thus many remain ashamed and unwilling to admit their troubles.

People with mood disorders benefit from the psychotherapeutic exploration of early childhood deprivations and abuse, but they do not magically recover as a result of this work. In fact, the depression itself operates selectively, causing sufferers to focus on past physical and emotional deprivation and abuse. While the early hurts contribute to the present illness, the current depression blackens the memories and strengthens their effect. Going over these past wrongs, whether real or imagined, does not make the depression go away. Sometimes it even deepens it. This is not a condemnation of the exploration of childhood in psychotherapy, which can be very valuable in terms of identifying the adult's emotional scars and dysfunctional patterns; rather, it is a caution regarding its efficacy in relieving major depressive illness. Most depression experts concur that the psychotherapy of depression must be of a different type from the exploration of childhood.

Should You Try One
of the Antidepressants?

Because depression can destroy a sufferer's hope for treatment of any kind, and can mire the person down with fatigue and indecision, and because this disease can also distort reality so he believes the suffering is deserved and should not be relieved, and because the illness may worsen gradually over months so that the individual is unaware that he rarely speaks, has lost the capacity for spontaneous activity, and no longer smiles, it is frequently necessary that the opinions of those who know the person be sought. While the list of depressive symptoms will aid a patient's self-diagnosis, the observations of friends, family, and trusted colleagues can help the individual decide whether to seek treatment. By the time the observations of those closest might be most valuable, they may have become angry with the patient, because many depressed people are very needy. They wear out their spouses and relatives with their angry, clingy behavior. It is essential that the depressed person pick someone whose objective description is not motivated by anger. If this person or several people all concur that the depressed person seems changed, down, not his or her normal self, then this is further reason to consider one of the antidepressants.

The next two steps involve the family physician, and then the expert psychiatrist or psychopharmacologist. That is because many medical diseases mimic psychiatric ones. The opposite is also true. Thus, psychiatric patients go to medical offices complaining of aches and pains caused by their emotional conditions, while those with unsuspected medical illnesses may be erroneously referred to psychiatrists. Unfortunately, most primary care physicians have neither the time nor, in many cases, the knowledge to deal with the complexities of psychiatric illness. It is the expert psychiatrist or psychopharmacologist who must be consulted for his or her knowledge of both medical and psychiatric conditions; which are which; how to manage the two at the same time; and how to factor in the occupation, social, and family aspects of the patient's life.

If you are not sure whether you or a loved one has a major depressive disorder, or wonder if it might be some other form of depression, or suspect there is something wrong but are reluctant to seek help, here are some ways to think about the decision.

You Have Tried to Help Yourself and Failed.

There is a lot of help out there, and some of the people I have seen have tried a fair amount of it, from diet to exercise, vitamins to vacations, workshop weekends to religious retreats, gurus to face-lifts, career change to spouse change, a new hobby, and mind control, and some or all have worked for a little while, and then no longer. Eventually, such attempts at self-help are abandoned because the person becomes discouraged, begins to believe nothing will help, and gives up. If the individual then sinks into the symptoms of depression I have already described, then such a person is a candidate for psychopharmacological evaluation, and perhaps one of the antidepressants. This decision should not be made in five minutes by matching a list of symptoms to those of major depression, but by a detailed and careful examination.

Psychotherapy Alone Has Failed.

Barbara began therapy when her six-year marriage started to fail. She wanted children and finally decided that Charles, her thirty-six-year-old husband, was more likely to act like a child himself than to father one. After much discussion, they agreed to separate and divorce. She felt she would never marry again, considered having a child anyway, but could not see how she could manage alone on the salary from her job at an insurance company. She found no one to date, withdrew from friends, and derived no pleasure from each day. She lost weight, had no interest in sex, and dragged herself to work.

All day she only looked forward to getting home, having several glasses of wine, and watching TV. She had no energy for phone conversations and refused the few offers her friends made, and soon they began to call less and less.

Barbara's therapy did not halt her decline. Rehashing her childhood seemed an academic exercise, and exhortations to make phone calls, see friends, and keep in touch with her family not only did not improve her situation, they made her feel worse. She liked her therapist, found her kind and well-meaning, even competent, but it was clear to Barbara that she was getting worse, not better. Her sister called her one day and recommended that she see a psychiatrist skilled in the administering of antidepressants. At first she snapped at her sister, but slowly she began to wonder if perhaps she was right. She got a referral and decided to see a psychopharmacologist.

Your Temper and Irritability Are Harming You and Your Loved Ones.

Joe and his wife have been married for twenty years. She does everything—taking care of him and the kids, doing the cooking, planning their active social life, and in addition, her earnings amount to half their income. Without her, the phone would not ring, no meals would be cooked, and the children's busy schedules would be in disarray. In spite of all her efforts, Joe criticizes her constantly, shouts at her unmercifully whenever she makes a real or imagined mistake, blames her for any money shortage or problem with the children. His temper has gotten so bad that his wife has begun to speak of it to her minister and to her close friends. Joe's attempts to calm himself with alcohol only make him worse. He is not a nice drunk. One of his wife's friends recommends psychiatric help and she says something to Joe. Naturally, he screams louder.

Antidepressant drugs calm rages and smooth tempers. These are not official uses of them—they are intended only for major depression—but they are nonetheless widely prescribed for this purpose, and they work effectively. Persuading Joe to go to a psychiatrist will require mobilization of his friends and family, and perhaps assistance from the minister and the family doctor. His wife may even have to threaten to leave. She is determined that he get psychiatric help, because living with him has become a nightmare.

You Have Low Self-Esteem.

The subject of low self-esteem could occupy this whole book, and certainly has in the case of many others. It refers to a chronic low opinion of the self to which the person is so accustomed that he or she does not consider it an illness. People with low self-esteem hide in bad jobs and bad relationships, convinced not only that they deserve no better but that if they were discovered, they would lose the little they have. By hiding in a job, I mean they do their work, take no chances, never complain, and hope the boss will leave them alone. Were they to be found out, they fear they would certainly be fired, since they consider their performance and themselves inadequate. The same is true of their marriage. They allow themselves to be badly treated by their families and friends because they believe themselves inadequate. Such people tend to be poorly paid, to be overlooked for promotion, to feel mistreated by their spouses and children, and to expect no relief. In fact, they have no hope that anything can change for the better.

You Have Chronic Pain.

Your chronic pain may be located in your head (headache, migraine), stomach or bowel, or in your back, and nothing you have done in the past has found its cause or cure. A trial on an antidepressant may provide the answer to your difficulties.

You Have Insomnia.

Insomnia is a complex and widespread problem. Especially when there is a depressed pattern involving difficulty falling asleep, frequent awakenings, and early-morning awakening, an antidepressant medication may prove very helpful, even in the absence of full depression. So may a hypnotic (a drug that induces sleep).

You Have Chronic Fatigue Syndrome.

In the nineteenth century, those who took to their beds in the absence of a clear medical reason were considered neurasthenic. This was sometimes an unfair attribution, because the medical cause existed but remained undetected. Presently, there are a number of people with chronic fatigue syndrome who are not suffering from a viral disorder or an undiscovered medical one, but who do not meet the criteria for major depressive disorder. These patients may respond to an antidepressant medication, and deserve a trial of one.

You Have Bulimia.

Those who are bulimic may respond to an antidepressant. Family studies have revealed a high rate of major affective disorder in the relatives of bulimics. Bulimia refers to recurrent episodes of binge eating followed by a compensatory effort to prevent weight gain, such as by inducing vomiting or taking a laxative. Treatment usually involves a combination of cognitive, behavioral, and drug therapy.

You Have Panic Disorder.

Panic disorder is characterized by sudden attacks of overwhelming fear which are accompanied by a pounding heart and trouble catching one's breath. The person feels dizzy and becomes afraid they are about to die. The first panic attack may occur for no apparent reason, or may follow a serious illness or accident, loss of a loved one, separation from family, childbirth, a thyroid condition, or abuse of a drug like LSD, marijuana, or cocaine. Patients may be convinced they are having a heart attack or losing their sanity. Usually the attacks last no more than twenty minutes. Subsequent attacks occur unexpectedly and fairly often and seem to be associated with deep, rapid breathing. Small doses of the older antidepressants have been very effective in blocking panic attacks, but not the fearful anticipation of them. Low doses of Prozac and other antidepressants and antianxiety agents have also been effective. Treatment takes three to ten weeks to work and must be continued for at least six months, but many patients require longer-term medication.

What Are the Types of Depression?

Major depressive disorder (MDD) is characterized by one or more major depressive episodes. These episodes, as previously described, consist of at least two weeks of depressed mood or loss of interest plus five of nine other symptoms of depression and no manic or hypomanic episodes. In addition, the depressive moods should not be due to substance abuse, a general medical condition, or schizophrenia.

Dysthymic disorder (dysthymia) refers to a depressed mood lasting at least two years, accompanied by two or more of the following symptoms: poor appetite (or overeating), insomnia or excessive sleeping, low energy or fatigue, low self-esteem, poor concentration or difficulty making decisions, and feelings of hopelessness. If a person has had a major depressive episode within the past two years, then the diagnosis becomes major depressive episode in partial remission rather than dysthymia. The diagnosis of dysthymia is also not appropriate if the patient has ever been manic or hypomanic or chronically schizophrenic or if the condition is due to substance abuse or a general medical condition. Furthermore, the symptoms must cause significant distress or impairment in social, occupational, or other areas of functioning. Dysthymic disorder can begin in childhood, adolescence, or early adult life, and is chronic in nature.

Dysthymia, also referred to as chronic mild depression, has

defied psychiatrists' efforts to define it. In the past, it was called depressive neurosis. The condition lies between major depression and the normal. When an individual has felt sad, hopeless, worried, gloomy, pessimistic, quick to take offense, easily hurt, and discouraged since childhood, she becomes accustomed to it. Depending on her beliefs, she may think life is not easy, rather than that she is ill. When Thomas Hobbes described the life of man in a state of nature as "solitary, poor, nasty, brutish, and short," was he doing so as a philosopher or a dysthymic? Are we to regard the sunny optimist as healthy and the dark pessimist as sick? A patient is not considered dysthymic if there is a "real" reason for it, such as a general medical condition or schizophrenia, but how about the death of a parent at an early age, or continuous physical or emotional abuse? Should we also include poverty, war, imprisonment, and poor diet as reasons for chronic mild depression coupled with low self-esteem, fatigue, and insomnia? I am afraid that efforts to place dysthymia in the biological camp and outside the psychological one—in the area of the chemical and out of the experiential—are unconvincing to me. Yet there is no question that antidepressants can sometimes treat this condition more effectively than psychotherapy. Just because a drug is effective in treating a psychiatric condition does not make its etiology hereditary or chemical. We are all ultimately composed of chemicals. If a lion were to walk into my office, the chemistry of my body and that of my patient would immediately change radically. If you did not know about the lion, but only measured the elements of the blood, you might think a chemical imbalance existed, when, in fact, the cause was fear of the lion.

Major Depressive Disorder: Will You Get Sick Again?

In over half the cases, MDD is a recurring illness. This is something that those who are not expert in the study and treatment of depression may forget. That is why it is necessary to obtain a careful history of a person's life. What was he like before he became depressed? Was he optimistic, productive, functioning well in work and outside, or was he dysthymic, gloomy, withdrawn, and chronically depressed? Is this the first or one of several episodes, and is there any pattern to what brings them on? One first-year graduate student came to my office because he found it very difficult to go to class and do his work. He wondered if perhaps he just did not want to become an economist and perhaps should have gotten a job after college and not sought a graduate degree. It was tempting to enter fully into a discussion with him of the pros and cons of economics, the dismal science, and of job prospects post-Ph.D., which also seemed dismal. But instead of prematurely beginning psychotherapy, I did as I usually do and took a careful history. His first year in college had also been very shaky. In fact, he had dropped out, gotten a job, and gone back to school, enrolling at an institution nearer to his close family. He went home each weekend, his laundry in tow, for a good meal and long talks with his mother. His first year of high school was also stressful, as he tried to fit in with a new group of classmates. He wondered if the others accepted him, and he felt especially awkward with girls. His grades initially suffered, but he was able to pull them up. It became clear that he was suffering his third depression, each brought on by the stress associated with transferring to a new school and separation from his close-knit family. The problem was not in economic graduate school, it was in him. First his mood needed to be improved, and then he could decide whether to continue. It was clear he had a mild form of an MDD: he took less interest and pleasure in his studies, had trouble sleeping, appeared tense and agitated, lacked energy, was unable to concentrate on his work, and had little hope for the future. Six weeks later, on 20 mg of Paxil daily, he was attending classes with interest and beginning to make friends. He continued to wonder if he should content himself with an M.A. in economics and then go to work, or stay on for a Ph.D. All his problems, including his excessive dependence on his family, had not been solved by Paxil, but he now had the energy to face them.

The course of MDD varies: there are otherwise healthy individuals who have a single episode and those who have many episodes; there are those who are asymptomatic between attacks and others who only partially recover, as well as some who never do. About 20 percent of major depression sufferers become chronic and remain partly or completely incapacitated by the disease. It is the physician's job to study the pattern of the illness and to vigorously treat it in order to prevent, or at least minimize, incapacity. Prompt, vigorous dosage of the proper antidepressant alone, or in combination with another medication, plus suitable psychotherapy, can rehabilitate the patient and allow him to lead a full, productive life.

Depression and Mania

Now called bipolar disorder, manic-depressive illness can severely disrupt a person's life. I will discuss the relationship between major depression and bipolar disorder, but a full description of this serious illness would require an additional volume. Nonetheless, it is necessary to pay it some attention because some major depressives evolve into bipolars, and because all antidepressant medications carry the potential for converting depression into mania.

Manic Episode

A manic episode is characterized by a persistent elevated or irritable mood lasting more than one week and accompanied by inflated self-esteem, decreased need for sleep, rapid speech, distractibility, racing thoughts, and participation in many risky activities leading to painful consequences. Manic individuals embark on an array of actions, often completing none. They are restless and get involved in buying sprees, imprudent business ventures, and unusual sexual activities, even with strangers. The disturbance is severe enough that the patient requires protection from the negative consequences of his poor business, sexual, illegal, or assaultive behavior. The symptoms of a manic episode may be caused by antidepressant medication, shock therapy, or drugs like corticosteroids. When drug-caused, the manic episode is not diagnosed as Bipolar I Disorder (also known as manic depression), but as Substance-Induced Mood Disorder with Manic Features. Patients during a manic episode usually do not recognize that something is wrong and consequently resist treatment. The patient may dress bizarrely, travel impulsively, become sexually aggressive, and engage in giving unsolicited advice to strangers. Ethical concerns may be disregarded and the patient may become assaultive. His or her poor judgment and excessive activity can lead to brushes with the law or large monetary losses. The patient's mood may rapidly shift to anger or depression. The patient may use large amounts of drugs or alcohol. Depressive symptoms are usually brief, lasting minutes or hours. If manic and depressive symptoms are significantly present every day for a week, the condition is considered Bipolar I, mixed type.

The first manic episode usually occurs between the ages of twenty and twenty-five, and begins suddenly with a rapid increase over a few days. Mania lasts several weeks or months, and the episodes are shorter than those of major depression. A major depressive episode often immediately precedes or follows a manic one.

Hypomanic Episode

A hypomanic episode is one in which an elevated, expansive, or irritable mood lasts at least four days and is accompanied by any three of the following: inflated self-esteem, grandiosity, little need for sleep, rapid speech, racing thoughts, distractibility, excessive involvement in activities and pleasures. Whereas manic episodes may be accompanied by delusions and hallucinations, hypomanic ones are not. To be considered hypomanic, the mood must be clearly different from the person's usual one, but not severe enough to completely disrupt work or social activities or require hospitalization. When there is a known cause for the manic or hypomanic episode, such as hyperthyroidism or an antidepressant medication, the patient is considered not to be bipolar, but to have manic features due to the medical condition or drug.

The hypomanic's mood is cheerful and unusually high, but may switch to irritability, and his or her speech may be filled with jokes and puns.

Bipolar I Disorder

To be considered Bipolar I (formerly manic-depressive), a patient must have had at least one manic episode. About 15 percent of major depressives will become Bipolar I patients. Unlike MDD, which is more common in women, Bipolar I Disorder affects men and women equally. Ninety percent of those having a single manic episode have subsequent ones, and about two thirds of manic episodes occur just before or after a major depressive one. Untreated, patients have four episodes in ten years on average, and the interval decreases as the patient gets older. About 10 percent of Bipolar I patients have four episodes of mood disorder (major depressive, manic, mixed, or hypomanic) per year, and these are called rapid cyclers. Most Bipolar I patients are normal between episodes, but about 20 percent are not. While studies show evidence of genetic influence in Bipolar I Disorder, it should be remembered that the large majority of individuals with Bipolar I close relatives do not become Bipolar I themselves. Bipolar disorders constitute 20 percent of all major mood disorders. Most bipolar disorders are treated with either lithium, Depakote (valproic acid), Tegretol (carbamazepine), an antipsychotic (e.g., Zyprexa) or antianxiety drug (e.g., Klonopin) for the manic phase, and an antidepressant for the depressed phase. Depakote (valproic acid) and Tegretol (carbamazepine) are anticonvulsants effective for acute mania and the prevention of relapses. Two new anticonvulsants, gabapentin (Neurontin) and lamotrigine (Lamictal), have been used to treat depression and mania in some treatment-resistant patients, as well as for other mood and anxiety disorders and to relieve pain. More studies will be required to establish whether Neurontin and Lamictal are good mood stabilizers. The best researched drug for bipolar disorder remains lithium, but Depakote is a close second and gaining.

Bipolar II Disorder

People who suffer hypomanic and major depressive episodes but may only remember and be troubled by their downs, and not by their highs, have Bipolar II Disorder. It is often their friends and relatives who identify the periods of elevated or irritable mood, rapid speech, lack of sleep, distractibility, buying sprees, sexual indiscretions, and foolish investments. The frequency of Bipolar II episodes is the same as that of Bipolar I.

It is important to distinguish bipolar from unipolar (episodes of depression only, no mania or hypomania) because it influences which drugs a patient should be given. The unsuspected Bipolar II can be tipped over into mania or hypomania by an antidepressant drug. Diagnosis is not merely an exercise in naming; it involves an assessment as to what is likely to happen in the future and how the patient should be treated.

Cyclothymic Disorder

An individual is considered cyclothymic if he has chronic mood swings that are not severe enough to constitute major depression or full mania. The mood swings must interfere with important parts of the patient's life, making him moody and unpredictable. Cyclothymic disorder usually begins in adolescence, and may go on to become Bipolar I or II Disorder.

Mild hypomania and mild depression are hard to distinguish from normal behavior. Whether an individual is merely moody or cyclothymic can be hard to decide, but the distinction is clearer if an attempt is made to judge whether the episode represents a change "uncharacteristic of the person when not symptomatic" (*Diagnostic and Statistical Manual of Mental Disorders*, 4th ed., 1994). Lithium and other mood-stabilizing drugs are as effective in cyclothymics as they are in bipolar patients. The cyclothymic patients who find their periods of hypomania productive and their depressions tolerable do not need mood-stabilizing medications.

What Causes Depression?

In *The American Psychiatric Press Textbook of Psychiatry* (3rd ed., 1999), the causes of depression are listed under three main headings—biological, psychological, and genetic—and under each of these are a half dozen or more models and theories. This textbook begins its discussion of the causes of major depressive disorder and bipolar disorder by saying they are "unknown" and that "a thoroughly satisfying explanation for the effectiveness of treatments is lacking." In clinical practice, I primarily find patients who fit each of the main textbook headings, and believe that the cause is biological, psychological, or hereditary. I believe that many of these people are correct in their estimate of the cause of their own depression. One woman insisted her depression was caused by the fact that she no longer loved her husband but could not divorce him because of the children. She refused to take an antidepressant drug. A salesman saw no reason to talk about his problems. He had heard that Prozac was very effective and wanted to try it. Then he would have renewed confidence and be able to go out on sales calls. The mother believed her depression to be psychologically caused, and the salesman biologically. Since there is an interplay between the inner biological state and the world outside, it makes sense that for one person, life events can be the main source of depression, and for another, bodily chemistry.

The genetic link for depression is stronger for people with bipolar disorder than for those with unipolar (major depression only) disorder. The incidence of mood disorder in relatives of unipolar patients is twice the rate in relatives of people without mood disorder, which translates to 10 percent versus 5 percent. This is a significant, but not overwhelming, association, which means that the relatives of unipolar patients are far from certain to get the disease. The hereditary line in bipolar disorder is much stronger, with about 25 percent of the relatives of a bipolar patient being either bipolar or unipolar.

The Biochemical (Neurotransmitter) Theory

Neurotransmitters are chemical substances that cross the gap from one nerve cell to the next (called the synapse) in order to stimulate or inhibit that cell. Originally, it was thought that too much of the neurotransmitters norepinephrine and serotonin caused mania, and too little caused depression. But because it could not be consistently shown that depressives had too little serotonin and norepinephrine, and because there was a several-week lag between the time these neurotransmitters were increased by antidepressant drugs and the first signs of clinical improvement, other explanations became necessary. Research attention has shifted from the synapse to the interior of the nerve cell to account for the time lag.

Other theories accounting for depression include hormonal abnormalities, such as low thyroid activity (hypothyroid) accounting for depression and an overactive thyroid (hyperthyroid) accounting for mania. Those depressives who do not get better on antidepressants may improve when thyroid medication is added. Another hormonal abnormality postulated is excessive corticotropin-releasing factor (CRF) by the hypothalmus, and new drugs to block CRF hold hope as antidepressants.

Psychological Theories

Psychoanalytic theories of depression emphasize the loss of love or status by a person made excessively vulnerable by extraordinary frustrations (or dissatisfactions) in childhood. Susceptible individuals made overly dependent because of early trauma react to a loss with the feeling that all is gone and the world is now empty. Their self-esteem severely diminished, they feel they are no good and no one loves them. Early deprivations made these people needy and angry and predispose them to depression. In psychoanalytic theory, frustration makes the vulnerable angry and the anger turns inward, causing depression.

Dr. Aaron Beck is a psychiatrist who devised the theory of cognitive behavior. Beck's theory is that depression (and other psychological problems) are caused by the way one thinks. Beck believes that depression is caused by negative views of the self, the environment, and the future which have been learned during childhood and adolescence. Dr. Beck has devised an effective psychotherapy of depression which teaches how to identify negative thinking patterns and how to reverse them.

The relationship of depression to life events can be difficult to establish. For example, did the patient become depressed because she was divorced, or was she divorced because she was depressed? Studies of the effect of a parent's death in early childhood as a cause of later depression show this to be an important event, but not as powerful as some psychoanalysts suggest. Stresses such as the death of, separation from, or strife with important people in the patient's life or failures and disappointments are more important in first episodes of depression than in later ones. The later episodes of depression are more easily elicited by weaker and weaker stresses once the initial pattern has been set, until it may become difficult to identify any trauma causing a relapse.

A Combination Theory
of the Cause of Depression

Two veterans of the horrors of war come home having had almost identical experiences. One is hospitalized with posttraumatic stress disorder and relives his terror in flashbacks, while the other prospers in his new job. Why the difference? There is an interaction of life events and the makeup of the person to whom they happen. This makeup consists of heredity and environment, both of which shape the individual who experiences the trauma. That is why the early death of a parent does not inevitably lead to depression. It depends on the child's heredity, life experiences prior to the death, and what happens afterward. This after-experience can be seen in the effect of divorce on children. It has been shown that if both parents maintain positive contact with the child afterward, the damage of divorce is minimized.

There are more than a dozen different types of depression. In addition, the fate of patients within a depressive category varies dramatically. This is well known in physical medicine, where one victim may die of a heart attack, and another live thirty years longer, where one arthritic person may complain of aches and pains, and another cannot walk. Similarly, one patient may become depressed after being fired from a job, but will snap back, while another will take to her bed for a year. Studies of abortion show that while most women are upset by it, only those with a tendency to succumb to stress become emotionally ill. Why some are vulnerable to stress and others possess the capacity for resilience is not understood. Insofar as a person's vulnerabilities are unique to the individual, each person must study his or her own, sometimes with the aid of a psychiatrist or psychotherapist, in order to learn to resist them better and bounce back faster.

It remains hard to explain why depressions often occur spontaneously and then disappear completely after about six months. If there is a biochemical abnormality, then why does it come and go? If it has something to do with serotonin, then why would the serotonin system go out of balance and then back in balance? Much progress has been made in the understanding of this terrible affliction, but the puzzle remains.

Why Are the Anxiety Disorders Included in This Third Edition?

Anxiety disorders were omitted as a distinct category from my first two editions, in what turns out to be an excessive focus on depression, fostered by the enthusiasm prevailing due to the introduction of Prozac (fluoxetine) in 1987 and earlier by that of Tofranil (imipramine) in 1958. In fact, the partitioning of anxiety and depression in psychiatric nomenclature antedates both drugs. It is true that these two occasionally exist in pure form, but this seems to be the exception rather than the rule. Depression and anxiety occur as symptoms in many psychiatric conditions, including schizophrenia, but are rarely diagnosed in those who suffer more dramatic disorders, such as psychosis or dementia. Feelings of anxiety and depression occur in everyone. The problem is when to define them as a disorder, a decision based on severity, duration, causation, and consideration of accompanying symptoms. Unfortunately, for those who try to define them, psychiatric syndromes are unstable. A person who has one at present next year may have another. A look at the thick charts of the severely mentally ill reveals a long list of psychiatric labels, influenced by how the patient presents at the time, and by whatever diagnostic system or treatment is available at the moment. An example of the latter occurred in 1970 when a large number of schizophrenics were reclassified as bipolar because lithium had become available. As you probably know, lithium is effective in bipolar patients and much less so in schizophrenics. In the mid-1950s, with the advent of the antipsychotic Thorazine, treatment by this drug was initially confined to hospitalized schizophrenics, but gradually spread to include a large number of nonpsychotics. Only when the dangers of Thorazine surfaced seven years later (tardive dyskinesia, a permanent movement disorder primarily of the face) did the usage of the drug become again limited to those for whom the indication was compelling. There was a somewhat different occurrence with Prozac. At

the time of its introduction, the manufacturer, Eli Lilly, responding to the lax use of this new "miracle" drug, recommended it
be prescribed only for MDD. Because, except for a minority
of psychiatrists who still insist Prozac is toxic, no severe univers-
ally apparent toxicity later surfaced, the widespread prescription in non-MDD patients remains. Part of this expansion
is to the anxiety disorders. It is a curious fact, I believe, that
no psychiatrist I know of has done systematic research on
whether the antidepressants are in fact safer than the original
benzodiazepine antianxiety agents in the treatment of anxiety
disorders, and few have tried to prove them more effective in
double-blind comparisons. Some treatments in psychiatry
merely go out of fashion. In fact, this was known to Sir
William Osler, who advised using a new drug "while it still has
the power to heal."

It has been said by a political wit that the Supreme Court's
decisions "follow the election returns" and one could make a
similar case that psychiatric diagnoses often follow the available treatments. Perhaps this practice will subside because of
the more rigorous *DSM* III of 1980. This new system may be
threatened, however, by the growth of psychiatric conditions,
which has become almost out of control. From 1968 (*DSM* II)
to the *DSM* IV in 1994, the number has proliferated from 159
to 357, and still more candidates for inclusion await the *DSM* V,
scheduled for publication in 2012. As a single drug, such as a
specific serotonin reuptake inhibitor (SSRI), is effective in
multiple conditions, some psychiatrists are beginning to question the therapeutic value of this expansion, and to suggest
either confining the *DSM* system to research only or reducing
the number of conditions for the clinician. I suspect that so
long as no objective criteria exist to establish and distinguish
one psychiatric disorder from another, the expert committees
will continue to meet and dream up more categories, or perhaps decide to reduce them, thus including only those relevant to specific treatments.

Generalized Anxiety Disorder (GAD)

In order to be classified as having GAD, the *DSM* IV requires excessive anxiety or worry for six months about various activities, such as work or school, which the person finds difficult to control. In addition, the anxiety and worry must be accompanied for six months by three of these six symptoms:

1. restlessness or feeling keyed up
2. being easily fatigued
3. difficulty concentrating (or the mind going blank)
4. irritability
5. muscle tension
6. sleep disturbance

These general symptoms are present in many settings rather than confined to certain situations, as the other anxiety disorders are, and must cause significant distress or impairment in social or occupational functioning. When other reasons exist causing the syndrome, such as drug or substance abuse, a medical condition, or another psychiatric disorder, then the name GAD is dropped. In summary, GAD is diagnosed when no other reason for it can be demonstrated. The line between those with a life-long anxious temperament and GAD requiring treatment is not clear.

The Overlap Between GAD and MDD

Both conditions:

1. cause sleep disturbance
2. cause fatigue and lack of energy
3. interfere with concentration
4. are responsible for gastrointestinal symptoms
5. can be associated with chronic pain, fear, apprehension, and worry

What Distinguishes the Two?

Anxiety disorders are associated with excessive alertness, abnormal fears of open or public places, or performance of rituals designed to reduce the feeling. MDD is more likely to be accompanied by low mood, loss of interest (as opposed to hypervigilance), and changes in weight and appetite. Both conditions take the pleasure out of living.

The main diagnostic difficulty is that the majority of GAD and MDD sufferers have both conditions, either simultaneously or alternately. In addition, they respond to the same treatments: drugs and psychotherapy. Furthermore, they improve after identical medications: Prozac, Celexa, Lexapro, Zoloft, Paxil, and Venlafaxine XR; the older tricyclic and tetracyclic antidepressants, such as Tofranil (imipramine), Elavil (amitriptyline), Norpramin (desipramine), and Asendin (amoxapine); the monoamine oxidase inhibitors (MAOIs), such as Nardil (phenelzine), Eldepryl (selegiline), and Parnate (tranylcypromine); the old barbiturates, and the benzodiazepines, such as Valium (diazepam), Klonopin (clonazepam), and Ativan (lorazepam).

The Other Anxiety Disorders

1. Panic Disorder (PD). This sudden attack of overwhelming anxiety accompanied by pounding heart, fear of fainting, choking, and death, has been mentioned in the section on MDD because of its frequent association with it. It also often overlaps with GAD (see pp. 80–81).

2. Phobia (agoraphobia, specific phobias). Agoraphobia is characterized by anxiety about places or situations which are associated with extreme fear and do not allow escape or access to help. The circumstances, such as being outside alone, on a bridge, or in an airplane are avoided, which limits travel, or causes marked distress when confronting the fear stimulant.

3. Social Anxiety Disorder (SAD). Anxiety is triggered by

contact with people, especially strangers, and by performance pressure, such as public speaking (see pp. 75–78).

4. Obsessive-Compulsive Disorder (OCD). Unwanted thoughts and repetitive behaviors designed to control fears which cause distress and interfere with functioning (see pp. 79–80).

5. Posttraumatic Stress Disorder (PTSD). The person experiences intense fear, amnesia, psychic numbing, or hyperarousal, following extreme trauma characterized by recurrent recollections of the event as if it were being relived, and tries to avoid situations that trigger reminders of it. Following the trauma, the person may experience PD, agoraphobia, SAD, MDD, and seek drugs or alcohol for relief.

All the anxiety disorders involve the excessive experience of anxiety, which is not associated with a specific cause in GAD, but is characterized by extreme episodes of panic in PD. Some psychiatrists believe PD ought not be a separate entity, because it is a severe, acute form of GAD. In SAD, the anxiety is caused by a social situation or the demands of a performance. In OCD, ritualistic behavior is engaged in to control the anxiety, caused by unacceptable thoughts or contact with parts of the environment considered germ-laden or otherwise dangerous.

Comorbidity

If psychiatric conditions are divided into narrow diagnostic categories, what inevitably happens is the phenomenon of comorbidity, which means in plain English having more than one of them, either at the same time, or following one another. Thus, the comorbidity of anxiety and depressive disorders is high, as is SAD and MDD, dysthymia and GAD, OCD and MDD (very high), PD with agoraphobia or simple phobia, both GAD and MDD together. The anxiety disorders frequently are comorbid with each other, making some psychiatrists wonder about the clinical value of subdividing them.

Before 1980, PD and SAD did not exist, but were subsumed within the anxiety disorder group. Now they are extremely common.

While it is true that people with many of the listed depressive and anxiety disorders have worse lives and functioning than those with only one of them, this may be a result of how severe the disorder is, or their reaction to it, rather than that they possess a long list of subdivisions within their category. Surely, for example, panic is more acute and troubling, accompanied by the fear of death, than is plain old worrying in long-term GAD. One does not have a worse prognosis because of comorbidity, but has comorbidity because of being sicker to begin with.

It is my view that the only diagnostic subgroups worth constructing are those that have a direct bearing on the treatment planned, unless one is doing research. If antidepressants are equally effective in anxiety, the division of the conditions is not worth it. If a specific phobia, such as fear of snakes, is not very responsive to drug treatment but is to the controlled exposure to snakes under a therapist's guidance, then the category makes clinical sense. As far as drug treatment is concerned, the development of specific drugs for well-defined psychiatric conditions remains a goal that has so far not been achieved. A statistical difference between two drugs for two conditions may look impressive on a graph, but may have little or no clinical significance.

Anger Disorders

No separate category in the *DSM* IV exists for anger, as it does for depression and anxiety, yet recent research reveals it to be as common a mood disorder. The failure to give it the equal status it deserves among these conditions has hampered diagnosis and treatment. In spite of the fact that depression and anxiety occur in many other psychiatric conditions, they have nonetheless been gathered together each in its own category. Anger, which also is spread among many psychiatric maladies, remains dispersed among them. This has resulted, for one thing, in no medications labeled anti-anger agents to go along with the antianxiety and antidepressant drugs. This does not mean that no thought or research has been done into anger and its treatment, but that it has been unfocused. The complete job of doing so here would require a separate volume, and thus I will confine myself to some general observations designed to help you decide if you are unduly hostile in your feelings or expressions, and how you might get some help from existing medications and a psychotherapist.

The Diagnosis of Disturbances of Anger

Psychiatry has traditionally divided its attention among feelings, thoughts, and behavior. This volume is primarily concerned with moods and feelings, but the separation in all cases is academic and artificial. I cannot conceive of a strong mood that is not accompanied by thoughts characteristic of it, and which does not affect behavior. This is true of anxiety and depression, and certainly is of anger.

People Are Much Less Likely to Voluntarily Seek Help with Anger Than with Anxiety and Depression

This may be one reason clinicians have been slower to recognize it. Many angry people experience their emotion as justified rather than evidence of a disorder for which they might seek help. The belief one is angry for good reason does not feel like a psychiatric problem, and too often it provides reason for direct action and remedy rather than evidence that one needs a drug or a therapist.

To make the assessment, even when the person comes for help with anxiety, depression, or some other reason, requires the diagnostician to specifically and gently inquire about its presence, and when it is denied, to look for it even when the person resists.

Some Reasons You Might Consider Getting Help for Anger

Anger can be a kind of primitive reflex that skips past consciousness and the civilized mind, and can easily result in thoughtless action when it is acute or in bodily damage when it is low level and chronic.

It might make sense to review your life problems and think about how an anger disorder might influence your thoughts, actions, and possibly your medical condition.

I have already noted that angry thoughts are usually experienced as justified by the actions of others, or by outside circumstances, and rarely as evidence of distorted thinking. You might try deducing whether you have an anger disorder by the consequences you suffer from it without realizing. For example, if you are frequently shouting at home at your spouse or children, it might be your short fuse rather than that they are being uniquely annoying. If you have lost several jobs or friends, it may be the fault lies in you. Try to discover whether there is any pattern in what triggers your rage, such as your spouse, boss, or perceived insults, so that you can learn to better control it. If someone else has spoken to you about your combativeness and temper, you might give their words some thought. If you break things or punch walls, you need to consider that you have a problem. If you have high blood pressure or bowel disturbances, you ought to examine your hostility level.

Irritable individuals are often impatient and intolerant of people around them, especially their family or fellow workers. The tendency to become easily annoyed can be kept inside, adding to anxiety, depression, health problems, and self-destructive acts, or externalized in the form of an explosive temper, argumentativeness, and damage to property. The effects of impatience, especially when not stifled, can damage one's career, children, marriage, and friendships, let alone result in confrontations with the law.

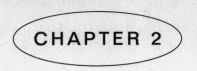

CHAPTER 2

What Are Antidepressants?

Antidepressants are drugs that are used to treat depression. They are often prescribed by general practitioners, psychiatrists, and by psychopharmacologists; the latter are medical psychiatrists who specialize in the study of the effects on behavior of drugs, as well as naturally occurring substances within the body, such as serotonin. Psychopharmacologists are keenly interested in the design and development of safer and more effective antidepressants. It is through their cooperation with research scientists at drug companies that the new, improved antidepressants were, and continue to be, developed.

Before these specialists existed, drug discovery depended entirely on serendipity. For example, the antituberculosis agent Iproniazid produced unexpected mood elevation in tuberculosis patients. Following up on this finding in 1957, scientists discovered that this drug did indeed have antidepressant efficacy in psychiatric patients. Thus, the first monoamine oxidase inhibitor was introduced to psychiatry.

In the early 1950s, the Swiss psychiatrist Roland Kuhn investigated several agents chemically similar to Thorazine, a drug that had just been discovered to be effective in the treatment of schizophrenia. He was looking for a treatment for depression, and after treating his first three cases in 1956, he discovered the first tricyclic antidepressant, imipramine (Tofranil), a close chemical cousin of Thorazine. John Cade, an unknown Australian psychiatrist who had no research training, was investigating the effect produced by injecting the urine of manic patients into guinea pigs. He chose to dissolve the urine's uric acid in water by combining it with lithium, the acid's most soluble salt. When injected into guinea pigs, lithium made the urine less toxic, so he became interested in studying lithium itself. He found that lithium carbonate injected into guinea pigs made them lethargic. Next, he tried lithium in ten manic patients in 1948 and found their excitement to be controlled.

In the last twenty years, antidepressants have begun to be designed based on neuroscience, rather than discovered by chance. Thus, cleaner drugs affecting only serotonin, norepinephrine, or both have been developed, producing many fewer side effects than the older antidepressants, which affected a variety of neurotransmitters, some of which were irrelevant to their clinical effect. Progress in designing new antidepressants is slow, because the brain contains about 10 billion cells, and more than fifty known neurotransmitters along with many unknown others, which influence many targets and produce varying effects on cell genes. In spite of this extraordinary complexity, progress is being made. Once the drug is designed, the gradual process of careful testing begins. It was fifteen years from the development of Prozac in 1972 by the scientists of Eli Lilly to its release by the U.S. Food and Drug Administration for public use in 1987.

In order for the FDA to allow the release of a new antidepressant, it must be safe and effective. Safety applies not only to the four to six weeks of a controlled clinical trial but to the long term. About 2,500 patients are given the investigational new agent and assessed for safety, but only several hundred of them are observed for more than a few months. The antidepressants nomifensine, bupropion (Wellbutrin), and zimelidine have been withdrawn from the U.S. market, although bupropion was rereleased with new prescribing instructions. Serzone has recently been withdrawn in Europe and Canada because of liver damage, but remains available in the United States. The safety of a drug must be carefully monitored after its release, not just before.

The effectiveness of any antidepressant is a complicated subject. The four- to six-week controlled trial compares the active agent to a placebo to show that the new drug is statistically superior. But this leaves two very important issues unaddressed. The first is an acute short-term one: that the difference between the drug and the placebo may be mathematically and statistically significant, but unimpressive clinically. That is, the patient may feel somewhat better—better than if he or she were on a sugar pill—but not completely well. Many psychopharmacologists have recommended that these trials be longer than the four to six weeks required by law so that the patients will have enough time to improve clinically, not just statistically. The second effectiveness issue is the long-term one. Does the improvement continue, or slip away? Is there a relapse in spite of the drug? Drug side effects that a patient notices or is willing to tolerate during acute deep depression may become intolerable in the long term. For example, the patient may not care about medication interfering with sexual functioning while deeply depressed, but he or she may stop taking the drug for this reason once he or she is feeling better. A drug that produces side effects of sufficient magnitude that patients stop taking it obviously loses its value. Since depression recurs in more than 50 percent of patients, the effectiveness of an antidepressant is very much influenced by a patient's willingness to remain on it.

What Is Improvement?

Full recovery may be used in reference to a person being totally asymptomatic, whereas *partial recovery* means that some symptoms remain, but not enough for the depression to be considered major. A *relapse* is defined as a return of symptoms during an ongoing treated episode. This happens when drug therapy is stopped too soon. *Recurrence* describes a new episode of major depression following the cure of a previous one. The importance of these distinctions, especially between relapse and recurrence, lies in deciding whether an acute episode has been treated long enough or whether the patient should be maintained on an antidepressant to prevent recurrence of new episodes.

Mood disorders have traditionally been thought to be episodic, with a good prognosis. This long-held view has been modified, however, by careful research. While the general outcome remains positive, 20 percent of major depressives are now believed to become chronic, 30 percent are unresponsive to antidepressant medication, and as many as 40-plus percent do not get well or are intolerant to the first drug tried. Half of these will respond to a second drug, and still more to innovative drug combinations.

While a total cure is the goal of every antidepressant drug treatment, it must be remembered that residual symptoms are all too common; they also imply a higher risk of relapse and prevent the depressed person from full participation in work and at home. Some estimates report total cures below 25 percent.

Three of the main rating scales used in evaluating new drugs in depression are the Hamilton, the global, and the Zung self-rating scales. The Hamilton is used in every study of a new antidepressant drug. It contains the following 17 items, and rates each on a 3- or a 5-point severity scale.

1. depressed mood
2. guilt

3. suicide
4. initial insomnia (difficulty falling asleep)
5. middle sleep insomnia (waking up in the middle of the night)
6. delayed insomnia (waking up too early and being unable to go back to sleep)
7. work and interests gone
8. retardation
9. agitation
10. anxiety—psychic (fearful thoughts, worry, tension, irritability, feeling jumpy)
11. anxiety—somatic (fast pulse, abdominal distress, frequent urination)
12. somatic symptoms—gastrointestinal (loss of appetite)
13. somatic symptoms—general (fatigue, muscle aches)
14. genital symptoms (loss of libido)
15. hypochondriasis
16. loss of insight
17. loss of weight

A total score indicates the number of symptoms and their severity. Severe depression is indicated by a score over 28, moderate depression between 14 and 28. Patients do not feel truly well until the score is under 6. In the four-week studies required by the FDA before antidepressants can be released, scores must fall by 50 percent for a drug to be considered effective. Typically, a drop from a Hamilton average of 24 to 12 occurs while the placebo fall is statistically significantly less, perhaps 24 to 15. At a Hamilton score of 12, the patient continues to feel badly. For this reason, many psychopharmacologists recommend that the trials be extended until the patients are completely recovered.

The Zung scale consists of a list of depressive symptoms which is self-administered by the patient and scored by the doctor. The global scale is the doctor's overall impression of the severity of the patient's condition.

Antidepressant Drugs Available in the United States

Generic Name	Brand Name
Monoamine Oxidase Inhibitors	
phenelzine	Nardil
tranylcypromine	Parnate
Heterocyclic Antidepressants	
imipramine	Tofranil, etc.
amitriptyline	Elavil, etc.
trimipramine	Surmontil
doxepin	Sinequan, etc.
amoxapine	Asendin
clomipramine	Anafranil
desipramine	Norpramin, etc.
nortriptyline	Pamelor
protriptyline	Vivactil
maprotiline	
Selective Serotonin Reuptake Inhibitors	
fluoxetine	Prozac
sertraline	Zoloft
paroxetine	Paxil
fluvoxamine	Luvox
citalopram	Celexa
escitalopram	Lexapro
Other Antidepressants (Unclassified)	
bupropion	Wellbutrin
trazodone	Desyrel, etc.
nefazodone	Serzone
venlafaxine	Effexor
mirtazapine	Remeron
duloxetine	Cymbalta

Monoamine Oxidase Inhibitors (MAOIs)

Monoamine oxidase inhibitors (MAOIs) are drugs that inhibit the enzyme monoamine oxidase from breaking down the neurotransmitters norepinephrine, serotonin, and dopamine and therefore cause the amount of each of them to rise. Nardil and Parnate are MAOIs that are effective in the treatment of major depression, especially so in atypical depression and also in bipolar depression. The main side effects of these drugs are sedation, dizziness, rapid heartbeat, insomnia, sexual dysfunction, constipation, and agitation. Their main disadvantage is the sudden severe elevation of blood pressure following intake of certain foods and medications. Patients cannot eat aged meats and cheeses and cannot take certain over-the-counter cold medications. The hypertension that may be induced can lead to headache, vomiting, palpitations, and occasionally to a stroke. Because of these side effects, necessitating dietary restrictions, MAOIs are typically not the first drugs used to treat depression. New, safer MAOIs are under investigation but so far have not been released.

Heterocyclic Antidepressants

Heterocyclic antidepressants (which include most tricyclics) were the most commonly used antidepressants for thirty years, given to millions of patients with excellent results. In fact, none of the new antidepressants are more effective than the 70 percent response rate achieved by these older agents. The selective serotonin reuptake inhibitors (SSRIs) like Prozac were developed because Elavil and Tofranil blocked serotonin reuptake, as well as that of norepinephrine, and it was hoped that the SSRIs would be as effective, yet less toxic. The tricyclic antidepressants (the term *tricyclic* refers to the chemical structure of drugs such as Elavil and Tofranil) have been used in many conditions other than depression. These include panic attacks, migraine, chronic pain, bedwetting, and bulimia. In addition, the older drugs were tested on hospitalized major depressives whereas the new SSRIs have mainly been researched in outpatients. Originally, it was believed that the more toxic tricyclic antidepressants might be more effective in the treatment of serious depressions requiring hospitalization. Their broad spectrum of action, affecting both norepinephrine and serotonin along with various other neurotransmitters responsible for their troublesome side effects, caused some to speculate that the inpatient and outpatient populations on whom the tricyclic and SSRI drug studies had been done were not comparable. Many wondered whether the Elavil- and Tofranil-like drugs might remain the drugs of choice for hospitalized depressives. This seems not to be the case, and many new studies have found the SSRIs to be equally effective in the treatment of severe depression.

It is not their effectiveness but the problems (discussed in the following section) associated with the older antidepressants that have caused their usage to decline.

Side Effects of Tricyclic Antidepressants

Heart and Circulatory

The tricyclics make the pulse speed up by 20 or more beats per minute. This can be frightening or annoying to people with healthy hearts and dangerous to those with a weakened cardiac status. The older antidepressants may disrupt the orderly beat of the heart, either by delaying electrical conduction within cardiac muscle, which can be seen on an electrocardiogram, or on rare occasions causing complete disorder and sudden death. The danger of sudden death is of particular concern in patients with serious heart disease and in children who are being treated with these agents in order to prevent bed-wetting. These drugs also may lower the blood pressure, especially in the elderly, who, when standing up after getting out of bed in the morning, may feel dizzy or lightheaded, and sometimes may fall and be injured. The tricyclics have been used safely for years, but now are avoided in favor of the newer antidepressants, especially in cardiac patients. When they must be used, the doctor should take a careful cardiac history, check the blood pressure and pulse, and evaluate the effects of other medical drugs being simultaneously taken; an electrocardiogram is advisable in older people before the tricyclic is prescribed. Follow-up cardiograms are necessary once maximum dosage has been established.

Visual

There are three main visual effects of the tricyclics. Some of the older drugs are worse than others on the eye. These drugs dry the eye and may be hazardous to contact-lens wearers. Artificial-tear preparations may help, but if the problem is severe, use of the drug may have to be stopped. Blurred vision is a second problem, which disturbs the individual's ability to read, especially early on in the treatment. Often this problem disappears after a week or two. The third problem can be avoided by a visit to the ophthalmologist to determine whether the patient has previously unsuspected narrow-angle glaucoma, in which case the older antidepressants pose a serious threat to eyesight and should not be used at all.

Gastrointestinal and Urinary

The older antidepressants are "dirty" drugs, meaning that they affect parts of the body not relevant to their therapeutic action. The same mechanism that dries the eyes also dries the mouth and slows the bowel and the flow of urine. Dry mouth occurs in some depressives not on medication and is worsened by tricyclics, while others experience this annoyance for the first time because of the drug. The effect may be reduced by sugarless lozenges or artificial saliva and often goes away by itself after several weeks, once the individual gets used to the drug. Sometimes dry mouth leads to tooth decay.

Constipation can be a symptom of depression and a side effect of the tricyclics. It can be mild and dealt with by dosage adjustment, fluid intake, or mild laxatives, but on rare occasions it can be severe, especially in older or medically vulnerable patients.

A slow urinary flow, especially in men with enlarged prostates, can be anything from an annoyance to an emergency when complete retention results.

When they are mild, the gastrointestinal and urinary problems are usually waited out in the hope that they will subside as the individual adjusts to the drug. If this does not happen, the dose may be reduced, or alternate antidepressants prescribed. Sometimes a drug such as bethanechol chloride (Urecholine) is successfully added to combat dry mouth, constipation, and urinary difficulties.

Weight Gain

Many patients who have been brought out of deep despair by the tricyclic antidepressants have stopped taking them because of a new misery—the effect on their weight. Some have gained as much as thirty pounds and risked falling back into depression rather than expand further. The reason for this added poundage is not entirely understood. It is not merely the return of pounds previously lost due to depression, nor is it due to swelling up because of water retention. Some investigators have described a carbohydrate craving stimulated by the medicine as well as a slowing of metabolism, but it is not known why this occurs. Some trycyclics such as desipramine and protriptyline seem to cause less weight gain and the Prozac-like SSRI drugs bupropion and nefazodone cause less weight gain, another reason why they are desirable. Unfortunately, weight gain is more common with Prozac and all the new antidepressants than was originally hoped.

Sexual Dysfunction

It is necessary to distinguish between those side effects caused by the medication and those caused by the illness itself. Loss of interest in sex is commonly experienced by depressed people who are not on medication. Before any antidepressant is prescribed this pattern must be carefully noted in order to evaluate any change. A person with a painful major depression may complain of many other, more troubling symptoms than loss of sex drive, which may not be mentioned at all. The thorough doctor will ask about sexual desire before prescribing an antidepressant. Then it is possible to differentiate between what is drug-induced and what is a component of the depression which has not yet been successfully treated. A person with major depression who feels better because of medication may begin to complain of loss of sex drive because preoccupation with suicide and the inability to work or care for the family present less of a problem. The remaining sexual difficulty can be caused by depression, prior inhibitions, relationship difficulties, or drugs. A careful evaluation before the drug treatment is started will help immeasurably in deciding the true cause.

Once the individual has fully improved, and it is determined that the tricyclic is to blame for impotence, lack of orgasm, loss of sexual interest, or inability to ejaculate, a decrease in tricyclic dosage may help without causing the person to relapse. If this fails, the antidepressant can be replaced by another one, or other drugs may be given to overcome the problem. Medications that can supplement the original antidepressant to overcome the drug-induced sexual difficulty are bethanechol or the antiserotonin drug cyproheptadine (taken an hour before intercourse to promote orgasm), yohimbine (to overcome impotence), and Viagra. These drugs are sometimes helpful but do not always provide the solution.

Suicide Potential

Major depressive disorder and bipolar disorder are serious illnesses with a fatality rate by suicide as high as 15 percent. Experts disagree regarding whether ideas of suicide are increased or stopped by the old or new antidepressants. However, there is no question that tricyclics were the leading cause of death by overdose in the United States. It takes only about a week's supply of a full therapeutic dose of Tofranil or Elavil for a patient to commit suicide. This sobering fact caused many family physicians to prescribe very low doses out of fear that patients would overdose. Thus, many depressives were inadequately treated by minuscule amounts of medication that in adequate dosage would have made them well. One great advantage of the new antidepressants is their much lower lethality. The tricyclics were found by one reviewer to be more than five times as likely to cause death by overdose as Prozac.

Similarities and Differences Among the New and Old Antidepressants

There is no difference in the cure rate among the antidepressant drugs now available, with the possible exception of the monoamine oxidase inhibitors Nardil and Parnate. If the other drugs are all equally effective in the approximately 70 percent of patients whose conditions they improve, then why were some experts reluctant to try the new ones? Many psychiatrists were at first a little slow in trying new agents that appeared safe but whose long-term toxicity was unknown. This attitude is not merely conservatism for its own sake. The long-term danger of the antipsychotic drug Thorazine was unknown until seven years after it was released. Abnormal movements of the face and tongue were noticed in patients who had been on the drug for more than six months, and as many as 20 percent of chronic hospitalized patients suffered this side effect. Worse still, it did not always go away when use of the drug was stopped, and sometimes it became worse. Although the initial report of tardive dyskinesia was published in 1959, seven years after the drug began to be prescribed, it was not until about five years later that the full extent of the problem became known. It was not uncommon in the 1950s and 1960s for Thorazine and its cousins (e.g., Stelazine) to be given in low doses to people who were not schizophrenic but merely nervous or unable to sleep. Physicians had no idea they were exposing people to the danger of developing these abnormal, permanent facial tics. Of course, a dozen years later, this became widely known, and the practice was stopped. I have spent all this time on Thorazine's late-occurring, unsuspected side effect to remind you that new drugs are not entirely without risk. And the problem with new drugs applies to the antidepressants. Nomifensine, a new antidepressant, was approved by the Food and Drug Administration in 1985 (only two years before Prozac) and then abruptly taken off the market because it attacked and destroyed red blood cells, causing severe anemia. Zimelidine, the first selective serotonin reuptake inhibitor (SSRI), was withdrawn in 1982 because in a small number of cases it caused sudden disease of the nerves leading to muscular weakness and paralysis. Fortunately, this does not seem to be a problem with the other SSRIs—Prozac, Paxil, Zoloft, Luvox, or Celexa. Finally, Wellbutrin was released by the FDA, then withdrawn because it was associated with a higher incidence of seizures than other antidepressants, and finally rereleased with more stringent dosage guidelines, which seems to have solved the problem. I cite all these mishaps not to excessively frighten you regarding new drugs but to underline the point that we do not know all there is to know about a drug when it is released, and if there are older, equally effective, safe ones, then continuing to use these rather than new ones with unknown dangers makes some sense.

The 70 Percent Improvement Rate

Seventy percent of all people taking antidepressants report an improvement, meaning that there is at least a 50 percent reduction in their symptoms. This is in comparison with 40 percent of people taking a placebo, whose symptoms of depression are also relieved. All the antidepressant drugs, new and old, achieve the 70 percent figure. What is not known is whether the various drugs improve the same 70 percent. The clinical suspicion is that different drugs help different patients, but doctors are unable to predict which individual depressed patient will be helped by a certain drug. It was initially thought that since the older antidepressants had been researched in sicker inpatients and the newer ones in less ill outpatients, each type would be most effective in the groups upon which they were tried. While this matter is being intensively researched, it appears that the new antidepressants are as effective in sicker inpatients as the older drugs are.

It is my belief that the new antidepressants do substantially better than the old ones in outpatient depressives. The reason for this is partly that they are better drugs, but mainly that they are being used more effectively. A doctor does not have to be an expert psychopharmacologist to use Prozac better than he used Elavil. Often when he prescribed Elavil he was afraid the patient would overdose, so very small doses were given in case the person took all of them at once. Since the typical family doctor did not see the depressed individual very often, he or she was in no position to trust the patient with a large supply of Elavil. The family doctor typically prescribed too little of the drug, and the patient did not recover. In the relatively rare case where the dosage was adequate, the general practitioner did not see the patient often enough to cope with the side effects, and the patient was likely to stop taking the medication. Only the psychiatrist or psychopharmacologist, who saw the patient more frequently, could encourage the acceptance of dry mouth, dizziness, blurred vision, constipation, and other unpleasant side effects while the dose was being raised to a point where it would be effective. The older antidepressants had dose ranges from one to twelve tablets and required careful increases, from a modest beginning to all twelve tablets in cases where the full amount was required. This rarely happened. Either the patient received too little of the drug or stopped taking the drug because of a side effect. In either case, he or she did not get better.

With many of the new antidepressants, patients require only one tablet a day. The family doctor does not have to carefully raise the dose until an effective level is reached. The drugs have a fairly low lethal potential so that the physician does not fear giving a month's supply at a time. Remember that one week's supply of Elavil could kill a patient.

Finally, the new antidepressants do not make patients faint or cause severe constipation, hand tremors, dry mouth, weight gain, or blurred vision. Because they are tolerated much better, patients do not stop taking them as often before they are successful at reducing symptoms. More patients are completing a full dose for an adequate period of time, are not discontinuing use of the drug against the doctor's advice, and are benefiting. The new drugs are thus doing a substantially better job in outpatient depressives, the majority of whom are being treated not by expert psychopharmacologists but by family doctors. The reason the new antidepressants have made such an impression is that they are easy to prescribe, are safe, can be given in full dose, and produce few side effects.

Remaining Problems

In spite of the great advance in the drug treatment of depression, three serious problems remain. These are the problems of lag time, treatment failures, and side effects.

Lag Time

If a person is severely depressed, preoccupied with suicide, unable to get out of bed, and experiencing difficulty at work or in caring for his or her family, there is a need for the individual to respond to treatment immediately, not after a week, a month, or half a year. In fact, a two-year follow-up study of 101 patients by Dr. Martin Keller et al. found that only 50 percent of these severely depressed people had recovered after one year. Patients with less severe symptoms have a better chance of recovery. The weeks or months of illness take a serious toll on marriage, work, family, and friendships, and increase the danger of suicide. Quick-acting antidepressant drugs must be found, but so far, in spite of claims by some company advertisements, no one medication has been proven to act faster than any other. Nonetheless, the situation is not all that bleak. Antidepressants markedly improve the condition of many patients within several days to a week, and double their chances for recovery within a month. They are among the most effective drugs, both in psychiatry and in all of medicine.

Treatment Failures

Without getting too technical, I must emphasize that there is a big difference between response and cure. A person who responds to a drug may be better able to function but may still suffer some symptoms. Someone who is cured is completely restored to health. While a degree of relief from symptoms is very important, the patient's overall ability to function may remain seriously impaired. It is necessary for the depressed patient to receive an adequate dose for a long enough period before being counted a treatment failure. Too often patients referred to university psychiatric facilities as drug-unresponsive have received inadequate dosages or the wrong medication. When treated properly, they then improve. Proper dosage is not a single standard, but varies from one person to another.

It has been estimated that 40 percent of those who have tried an antidepressant cannot tolerate the side effects or do not respond to the first drug with which they are treated. Of these, an additional 50 percent respond to a second antidepressant, perhaps more so if it is of a different type. Thus, someone who fails on an SSRI (like Prozac) might respond to Wellbutrin. This leaves 20 percent who fail to respond to the second drug. These people are given one of several drugs in addition to the second antidepressant, such as thyroid, lithium, a tricyclic (if the SSRI failed), buspirone, trazodone, Ritalin, or estrogen in women. Many of these combinations seem to work. There is little research evidence to prove this, however. Rather, the practice has clinical, anecdotal support. Controlled studies are necessary to establish that the observed improvement is due to the active drugs and not to the passage of time or the placebo effect of changing medicines. With these added drug treatments, over 90 percent eventually respond—a very fine result—but unfortunately, 5 or 10 percent do not.

Side Effects

The trouble with the older antidepressants was that many people could not tolerate them at all, or were unable to accept high enough doses to get the full benefit. As a result, many stopped taking them, or were maintained on such low amounts that they received little help. The physician had to repeatedly encourage patients to suffer more discomfort on the drug than their depression had made them experience in the first place, until one to three weeks had elapsed and they began to feel better. By this time, the side effects often subsided as the person became used to the medicine and felt better.

The new antidepressants are much better tolerated and represent a great advance. Nonetheless, about 15 to 20 percent of people who take them cannot stand the abdominal distress or "drugged" feeling, or other side effects, and must stop taking the medication. An equal number do not improve, so that the figure of about 40 or more percent who fail to improve on their first antidepressant remains. This situation is not unique to psychiatry. Many medical patients on blood pressure medication either cannot tolerate or fail to respond to the first drug tried. People who are depressed are in pain, and their ability to function is often hampered. It would be best if the doctor knew which type of depressed patient would respond to which drug, and could prescribe the correct one right away. But unfortunately, there is no way to predict this. The same is true for hypertension. There are many different drugs belonging to various drug classes, but the doctor cannot predict with certainty which one will be effective. It is important that anyone contemplating taking an antidepressant medication for the first time realize that there is a good chance the first drug might not work, and they should be prepared to try a different drug if necessary. Their chances of eventually being significantly helped are very good.

Treatment Response and Cure

Initially, it was hoped that Prozac could make depressed people better than well, or at least completely cure them. I have seen patients with chronic, lifelong mild to moderate depressions feel better than they could ever remember. I have seen acute major depressive disorder patients smile and joke again as a result of their antidepressant treatment. But I have seen a fair number of partial improvements, patients who are once again able to sleep, eat, work, and participate in family life, but who still take little or no pleasure in life. They drag themselves through the day and collapse in bed at night. The depression is lessened, controlled, but not gone. I believe this is the reason why new antidepressant drugs continue to find a market among those whom the older drugs have not fully cured. I also am convinced this is why depressed people should never be treated by drugs alone, because too often these agents do not cure the patient. The psychiatrist must carefully evaluate the sufferer's overall functioning rather than settle for partial improvement with continued impairment, which can be addressed through psychotherapy.

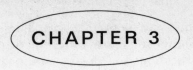

CHAPTER 3

The Selective Serotonin Reuptake Inhibitors (SSRIs): Prozac, Zoloft, Paxil, Luvox, Celexa, and Lexapro

Serotonin

Serotonin is one of the chemicals in the brain that transmits messages from one brain cell to another. It would be nice if the serotonin story were as simple as this: too little causes depression; too much, mania. But in fact, brain activities are controlled by the coming together of many different chemicals (also known as neurotransmitters), which serve as messengers from one cell to the next. Brain cells are excited not only by serotonin but also by norepinephrine, histamine, gamma-aminobutyric acid (GABA), and acetylcholine, to name just a few. The interactions of the fifty-odd neurotransmitters with serotonin, therefore, involve serotonin in many brain activities that are disturbed in psychiatric symptoms and disorders, such as depression, anxiety, irritability, confused thinking, abnormal appetite, and disturbance of the sleep cycle. Furthermore, the neurotransmitters affect one another, and that may be why serotonin and nonserotonin antidepressants work equally well—when you give a drug affecting one neurotransmitter, you automatically affect the other neurotransmitters.

The term SSRI refers to selective serotonin reuptake inhibitor, a class of antidepressant drugs that are safer than, yet equally effective as, the older tricyclics. The SSRIs have mainly been researched in patients suffering from pure major depression and, to a lesser extent, in those suffering from obsessive-compulsive disorder and bulimia. Nearly every day, however, there are clinical reports of their effectiveness in the treatment of yet another condition. This seems to support the notion that there is a serotonin imbalance which crosses disease categories and explains this wide-ranging response. Because the SSRIs are safe drugs, and because the conditions they treat are serious, clinical necessity has forced their use before firm evidence of their effectiveness could be established. Anecdotal reports keep pouring in: the first known case of this or that, of a seventy-five-year-old stroke victim who cried for no reason being successfully cured by Zoloft, of two violent patients with different psychiatric conditions becoming much less aggressive after Zoloft. Later, I will list all the conditions to which the SSRIs have been applied with reported success, but with as yet insufficient scientific evidence. I do not wish to imply that these clinical efforts are in any way irresponsible. Physicians do not have complete and final evidence for much of what they do, some of which is much more serious than the mere prescribing of an SSRI. The example of the radical mastectomy comes to mind. When I was at Columbia University's College of Physicians and Surgeons from 1955 to 1959, the great Cushman Hagenson said emphatically that radical mastectomy was the only operation that could give a woman with breast cancer a chance at a full cure. Today, we know this is not the case. It seems he did not have all the evidence.

The SSRIs as a Class

More than half of all new antidepressant prescriptions written in the United States are for SSRIs. In the previous chapter, I called attention to their ease of use and their greater safety as being primarily responsible for their popularity. Because patients tolerate SSRIs better than the older antidepressants, more are able to complete an adequate dosage trial for a sufficient period of time to gain the full benefit of medication. A 1995 study noted that 60 percent of the depressed are treated by general practitioners who spend little time with these patients. They will give them a month's supply of SSRI at a time, instruct them to take one a day, and not worry too much about lethal overdose or about complicated side effects leading to noncompliance. Patients take these SSRIs daily and get better. The general doctor need not pay too much attention to them. Of course, there is some danger in inadequate medical supervision. The patient could have an unsuspected bipolar illness and be tipped over into mania by the SSRI. Furthermore, a study by A. C. Pande and M. E. Sayler (1993) of 3,183 outpatients in nineteen controlled studies of Prozac compared with a placebo or an older antidepressant found a remission rate in the severely depressed of only 27 to 29 percent on Prozac, 26 percent on a tricyclic antidepressant, and 18 percent on a placebo. These results are far from spectacular and demonstrate the need for the physician to carefully follow severely depressed patients and not merely send them off with a Prozac prescription in the naive belief that they will all get better. Once again, I must remind you of the difference between response (about 70 percent) and cure (found in this study to be only 27 to 29 percent). The improvement rate in the mild to moderately depressed as well as the cure rate, a Hamilton Depression score of 7 or less (see the previous chapter regarding Hamilton scores), is much better than in the severely depressed. But it is still far from perfect. People who are depressed, no matter how severely, need to be monitored closely for dose adjustment when necessary, and the doctor should check their medical status and psychiatric improvement and offer words of explanation, encouragement, and psychotherapy along with the drug. It would be nice if the scourge of depression could be completely resolved by a simple pill, new or old, SSRI or not, but this is far from always the case.

Nonetheless, the problems with the serotonin theory and the shortcomings of the SSRIs aside, these drugs have been very effective in treating the typical outpatient depressive. Safe and well-tolerated, they are usually effective taken once a day, often only a single pill. It is worth considering them together as a class before looking at their individual differences because they have much more in common than they have differences.

The issue of classification of the twenty marketed antidepressants presents something of a problem. Some of the medicines are classified on the basis of their chemical structure (e.g., the tricyclics), some on the basis of their action on neurotransmitters (e.g., SSRIs), and some are not classified at all but listed simply as "other" (e.g., Wellbutrin). But in spite of this difficulty, it may make sense to use an antidepressant of a different class if the first one fails.

The SSRIs alter serotonin balance, but exactly what happens is not fully known. At first it was thought that by blocking reuptake they raised the level of available serotonin, but now it is known that the receptors are altered by becoming less sensitive. In any event, it is believed that serotonin is involved in the control of aggression, in sexual behavior, and in the maintenance of mood. The SSRIs, because of their effect on serotonin, have been used not only in depression but also in the following conditions:

Generalized anxiety disorder
Obsessive-compulsive disorder
Panic and other anxiety disorders
Bulimia and anorexia nervosa
Schizophrenia

Alcoholism
Borderline personality disorder
Autistic disorder
Impulsive aggressive behavior
Postpartum depression
Premenstrual syndrome
Social phobia
Pedophilia
Migraine headaches
Intermittent explosive disorder

According to the evidence, their effectiveness ranges from excellent in depression and anxiety, to reasonably good in obsessive-compulsive disorder, and anecdotal in many of the other conditions. I am sure this list of SSRI uses is incomplete. Every day something new is added.

The SSRI Cure

Karen Jones, a forty-year-old married mother of one, had been unhappy in her marriage to John, her cold and uncaring husband, for almost all of the seven years they had been together. Not only did he not help with their four-year-old daughter, he seemed to avoid both of them, coming home from work as late as possible and going off to his study to hide and read. Karen felt lonely, angry, and unappreciated. She never smiled at John, refused sex except on the rarest occasions, and complained bitterly to him about his coldness and lack of cooperation in their family life.

Karen slept poorly, and appeared tired and grim. She stopped planning their social life and no longer read novels, previously her favorite activity. Karen had been seeing a therapist for two years. Much of the time they discussed her unhappy marriage, but she seemed unable to improve it. John refused to come to see the therapist with her, and Karen realized she could not fix her marriage alone. Besides, how could a withdrawn, cold engineer be transformed into a loving husband and father? Karen continued to worsen. She remained longer and longer in bed, returning to it as soon as she dropped her daughter off at preschool. She slept badly at night, started to lose weight, and stopped speaking to her friends and family. Her therapist, having become alarmed, suggested a psychopharmacology consult. A diagnosis of major depressive disorder was made, and she was given a prescription for Prozac. She asked the doctor why an SSRI and why the particular one she was suggesting. Her doctor said that all antidepressants, old and new, had the same power to help her, that the newer ones had fewer side effects, and that of the ten newer ones, she had the most experience with the SSRIs. She decided to prescribe 10 mg of Prozac each morning, half the typical 20-mg starting dose, because some people could not tolerate the larger amount right away.

She added that the other SSRIs had some advantages. They were not as activating, so that people felt less "wired" and nervous on them, whereas dry mouth and drowsiness were more likely with Paxil. All the SSRIs cause insomnia, which can often be overcome by taking the drug in the morning or by lowering the dose. Nausea is also a problem with the SSRIs, which can be lessened by taking the medicine with meals and tends to disappear after several weeks. Common to all SSRIs and estimated to afflict between 30 and 40 percent (some experts say up to 80 percent) of users is sexual dysfunction in both men and women. The doctor went on to say that although the ten new antidepressants were all as effective as the twelve older ones and caused fewer side effects, none of them were perfect.

One week later, Karen returned for a follow-up visit, saying she was sleeping a little better, and she appeared less grim and tired. Otherwise, nothing had changed. She continued to spend too much time in bed. The psychopharmacologist asked about side effects and, discovering none, raised the Prozac dose to 20 mg. Two weeks later, on her return visit, Karen said she felt a little nervous and had a little diarrhea, but that neither was excessive. What had changed was that she was no longer spending the day in bed. In fact, she had been to lunch with several of her friends and had had a good time. She did not feel up to books yet, but had read several magazines and had gone to a lecture she enjoyed. On each of her biweekly visits over the next several months, she reported slow but steady improvement, until, after the fourth month of treatment, she told the psychopharmacologist something the doctor considered quite remarkable. Karen had had a talk with her husband in which she discovered he had been quite angry at her for what he perceived as her laziness and lack of attention to him and the child. His perception had been that he did all the work outside the home and then came back to do everything inside it as well. He was less angry now that Karen had gotten out of bed and begun to straighten up their home and their marriage. He enjoyed sex with her for the first time in years, in spite of his understanding that Prozac hampered her responsiveness. Most of all, John said, he felt once again, for the first time in years, that Karen loved rather than hated him, and he once again enjoyed being with her. Indeed, John began coming home earlier from work and enjoyed the company of his wife and daughter.

Karen reported that she understood the effect of her depression on her husband, how her lack of energy and anger had made him withdraw warily from her. She was fully aware that what she gave in her marriage was what she got; that if she was good to John, he would be kind to her. She also marveled at how this simple recognition had eluded her in her years of therapy. In fact, the sympathy of her therapist regarding how hard it was for her to be married to this cold, withdrawn man implied that he had caused her depression, rather than merely responding to and suffering because of it.

How Effective Are the SSRIs?

Every antidepressant treatment, including the SSRIs, older antidepressants, and even electroshock, affects serotonin neurotransmission. All the SSRIs are equal in efficacy to all the older and newer antidepressant drugs, but they have fewer side effects. The reason for this lies in the word *selective* in selective serotonin reuptake inhibitors. While the ability to tolerate SSRIs better than older antidepressants is of enormous importance, the hope that they would cure more patients has not been realized. In general, there is no one group of depressives or patients who benefit more from an SSRI than from other antidepressant drugs. Furthermore, the SSRIs do not cure patients more rapidly than other antidepressants. With all the antidepressants, there is a five-day to three-week or longer wait before improvement occurs.

The SSRIs have proven to be as effective as older antidepressants in the treatment of severe depression. Unfortunately, as I mentioned earlier, while the response rate in severe depression is not too bad, the cure rate is low and slow for the SSRIs. These are wonderful drugs, but they are not miracle drugs. Patients with severe depression must tolerate weeks and months of waiting before they truly feel better.

Of All the Antidepressants, Old and New, Should the SSRIs Be Used First?

Judging by the number of prescriptions written, most psychiatrists prescribe SSRIs first. The SSRIs are as effective as any of the others and have the fewest side effects. Most people tolerate them well and are able to complete a full course of treatment. They only have to be taken once a day, which is easy to remember. Most of the time, one pill is all that is needed, which makes frequent trips to the doctor for dose adjustment unnecessary. Because they have been prescribed so widely, many of their few bad secrets have been revealed. Brand-new drugs pose unknown risks.

The SSRIs are the antidepressants I use first, and often second, too, if the first one fails or cannot be tolerated. It is only then that I will turn to a newer or older agent. Most physicians seem to do the same.

Depression Combined with Anxiety

Many depressed patients also suffer from anxiety. Anxiety affects both mind and body, causing gloomy and fearful thoughts, along with rapid pulse, sweaty palms, and abdominal symptoms. Whether one causes the other or both are produced by something else is unknown. What is known is that a patient with a major depressive disorder is more than ten times as likely to develop an anxiety disorder either simultaneously or in the future. Perhaps this is further evidence for the serotonin or neurotransmitter imbalance I spoke of earlier, since serotonin may play a role in both anxiety and depression. It may be that it is irrelevant. If aspirin cures a headache, is the headache due to aspirin deficiency? Various theories notwithstanding, many physicians were concerned about prescribing an SSRI to depressed patients who were also anxious or prone to anxiety since one prominent side effect of these new medications is an increase in anxiety, especially early in treatment. These physicians reasoned that a sedating antidepressant such as Elavil or Paxil would be a better choice. This clinical "logic" has proven incorrect. Ironically, anxiety can be a side effect of the SSRIs, yet they are as good as many of the older sedating antidepressants in the treatment of anxiety accompanied by depression.

SSRIs are now being used effectively in every variety of anxiety disorder, including panic disorder, social phobia (also termed social anxiety disorder), obsessive-compulsive disorder, posttraumatic stress disorder, and most recently, generalized anxiety disorder. The SSRIs can just as accurately be called antianxiety agents as antidepressants. Because of this, they recently have been accepted formally by the FDA for the treatment of anxiety disorders.

Suicidal Preoccupation

Contrary to an early false report, the SSRIs do *not* cause or worsen suicidal thoughts or behavior. Unfortunately, as with all other antidepressants, SSRIs are not effective in 30 percent of patients, and the failure figure is higher in severe depressives. Suicidal thoughts and attempts occur during SSRI therapy at the same rate as they do during tricyclic antidepressant treatment, but overdose deaths are much lower from the new drugs than the old ones. When compared to a placebo, SSRIs lessen suicidal thoughts and actions. SSRIs are much safer if an overdose is taken than the tricyclic and MAOI antidepressants. However, any time more than seventy-five pills are ingested, serious effects on the heart, while rare, are nonetheless possible, and generalized convulsions are likely. In the two cases where death resulted, more than two hundred pills were swallowed. When taken in overdose, Prozac causes nausea, vomiting, and restlessness, and Zoloft and Paxil overdoses cause drowsiness and a slowed pulse rate. SSRIs are much safer for the heart than the older tricyclic antidepressants. Nonetheless, doses of SSRIs can slow cardiac conduction and induce rapid beating of the ventricles, a potentially dangerous combination.

Switches into Mania

Occasionally, a depressed person turns into a manic one. On the rare occasions when this happens, the consequences can be very serious and the patient may require hospitalization. When someone is a known bipolar (manic-depressive), this danger can be guarded against with medication. Sometimes, however, this occurs unexpectedly. The question of whether such events are caused by the antidepressant medication or whether the person was simply due to have a manic episode is difficult to settle in an individual instance. A few studies and several experts have found that the SSRIs are associated with manic switches in 1 percent of cases whereas the tricyclics are responsible in 2 percent. They recommend shorter-duration SSRIs like Paxil so that if the manic episode is induced, use of the drug can be stopped without lingering effects. Over the years, I have found the manic switch to be very rare in depressed outpatients without a history of mania or hypomania and who have no manic-depressive relatives. On the rare occasion when it does happen, it is best spotted by a friend, relative, or doctor since the patient may suffer a loss of judgment and be unaware of what is happening.

SSRIs are effective in known bipolar depressed people who are taking lithium, Tegretol, or Depakote. They may be used safely and in the normal dosage.

Dysthymic Disorder

Dys means "bad" and *thymia* means "mind" or "soul" in Latin. Dysthymic disorder lies on the border between the normal and the pathologic, and that border is engulfed in fog. The official psychiatric diagnostic manual has attempted to clear that fog three times in the last fourteen years (1980, 1987, 1994) without great success. The psychiatric microscope remains uncleaned and without power to tell us what is the normal level of suffering associated with the human condition and what is pathologic. It currently defines dysthymic disorder as a "chronically depressed mood" present for most of two years or longer, and accompanied by changes in appetite, sleep, and energy along with low self-esteem, poor concentration, difficulty making decisions, and feelings of hopelessness. An individual need have only two of the ten items listed in addition to a chronic bad mood, so many different combinations of symptoms are possible. For example, if someone feels sad and is overweight and without much energy, that person is dysthymic. Another individual may feel down, have difficulty concentrating at his job, and have low self-esteem. He, too, is dysthymic. Someone else may have trouble sleeping and making decisions and feel down in the dumps. She, too, is dysthymic. Another individual may sleep too much, eat too little, and feel depressed. The question of who has the illness dysthymic disorder, requiring a drug, and who is not sick but needs to change his life in order to feel better can be a difficult one for doctor and patient.

The concept of dysthymia and the efforts to objectively depict it arise out of a desire to make psychiatry scientifically valid and objectively capable of studying its illnesses and treatments. The observable symptom list of dysthymia replaces the concept of neurosis with its hidden, unconscious desires and conflicts, largely inferred by psychoanalytic believers and difficult to see for nonbelievers. Dysthymic patients are the "neurotics" of twenty years ago, and the people who now take care of them would like to be able to agree with one another regarding their diagnosis and treatment.

The problem for psychiatry is shared by all of medicine. There are the very sick, the well, and all those in the ill-defined middle. The cancer doctor has the same difficulty: he or she tries to grade cancer 1, 2, 3, 3b, 4, 4b, or 5, in order to tell what will happen to the patient or how long she will live. Grade 1 may be very slow-growing and grade 5 overwhelmingly fast, but the numbers in the middle may not mean much. Some dysthymics are quite dysfunctional, drag themselves to work if they are even able to do that, but otherwise lie in bed or sit on a couch. They have few social contacts, no hobbies or interests, and exist from day to day without goals or pleasure. The healthy dysthymics are lawyers or surgeons who work all the time, do not smile much, are over- or underweight, and may have trouble making decisions or falling asleep. Are they sick or merely grim? The sick dysthymics often have episodes of major depression. Do they have two diseases (so-called double depression) or is it a varying expression of the same illness? The healthy dysthymics continue on in their plodding, workaholic ways. The analogy with cancer grading applies—those with mild forms will probably die of something unrelated. The questions as to which cancerous prostates to remove and which to leave untreated until old age or some other condition leads to death continue to be debated. Almost all agree that something ought to be done about the severe cases of cancer, and similarly of dysthymia. A 1995 article published in the *American Journal of Psychiatry* adds to the complexity of dysthymia. The authors found that lifelong dysthymics are much more inclined than those people with episodic major depression to have borderline, histrionic, self-defeating, dependent, or avoidant personalities. The researchers refused to take a position on whether the personality disorder caused or was a result of the dysthymia, or whether both were due to some unknown reason. But the study once again shows the link between illness and personality and the difficulty of separating one from the other.

SSRIs help dysthymics, but almost all the evidence is anecdotal. These are the people who have been depressed since childhood, who Peter Kramer, author of *Listening to Prozac*, reported felt "better than well" on Prozac. Most psychopharmacologists and psychiatrists (including myself) think not that the drug gave them an artificial high, but that it removed their depressive features, allowing their self-esteem to rise, along with their energy and mood, so that they could function in a healthy way for the first time. Many of these people had been in psychotherapy for years with varying degrees of benefit, but Prozac made a profound difference. I have seen this phenomenon occur in my practice, sometimes after having worked with the person in psychotherapy without drugs for several years. An SSRI lifted the person's confidence, helped him organize his thoughts, gave him the courage to speak before a group, helped him become more active in the community, and brightened his outlook on life. Some who never expected anything good to ever happen began to plan optimistically.

The writings on dysthymia regarding drug treatment come mostly from those who have observed the sick end of the dysthymic spectrum, those who describe the frequency of major depressive episodes in this group. My own experience with outpatient, functioning dysthymics has made diagnosis much more difficult than it is for those who deal with the sickest end of the condition. On the healthier side, they are limited in their occupational, social, and family functioning, yet it is not so easy to say whether they are experiencing normal human suffering or dysthymic disorder. I tell such people about the SSRIs and explain that my capacity to guide them is limited. It is up to them to decide whether their suffering has gone beyond the edge of normal. Most decide to do without the drug. Of those who try, a large majority feel much better, and the quality of their lives improves. Occasionally, I run into a drug-type who will ingest anything for a new experience, or to achieve a high, but most of my patients are not that way. They are sincerely trying to help themselves and their friends and families. I trust these people to make their own diagnosis with the help of my limited knowledge.

I think it will be a long time before science will be able to define accurately and cure dysthymia. The condition is chronic, hard to diagnose, and frequently difficult to treat. The diagnostic criteria keep changing because of advancing knowledge, and the changes present a problem for the study of a chronic illness. Studies begun years ago are no longer valid for current purposes of diagnosis. This is particularly problematic for a vague condition like dysthymia, but even what I called schizophrenia during my residency in the early 1960s is no longer considered schizophrenia. Does this mean the drug studies of that era no longer apply?

I leave you with my conviction, shared by many of my colleagues, that if you suffer from dysthymia and it interferes with your work and your relationships with your children, friends, family, and lovers, and if therapy has helped to some extent, but not enough, try an SSRI. It could make a huge difference for you.

If Side Effects Force You to Stop One SSRI, Will You Be Able to Tolerate Another?

Drs. Walter Brown and Wilma Harrison questioned 113 patients with major depression (*Journal of Clinical Psychiatry*, January 1995) who had discontinued Prozac because of side effects. The side effects most commonly causing patients to stop taking the drug were insomnia, agitation, anxiety, headache, sleepiness, nervousness, fatigue, decreased libido, impaired concentration, and nausea. A month after stopping Prozac, they were started on Zoloft. Seventy-nine percent of the patients completed Zoloft treatment, and only 10 percent discontinued because of side effects. The patients completed several months of Zoloft treatment in spite of gastrointestinal symptoms, insomnia, sexual dysfunction, somnolence, and agitation. One shortcoming of this study is that it was not double-blind—that is, it did not give half of the patients Prozac again and the other half Zoloft without telling them which one they were getting. In spite of this, it seems to make the point that if one cannot tolerate Prozac, another SSRI may do. My personal clinical experience corroborates this fact. People who cannot tolerate one SSRI frequently respond well to another.

SSRI Use During Psychoanalysis

During my Harvard psychiatric residency more than forty years ago, one of my professors, Dr. Elvin Semrad, a legendary psychoanalytic teacher in Boston, required us to stop medicating our patients before he interviewed them so that their heads would not be disconnected from their bodies and he could discover what really bothered them—the feelings they found it so difficult or impossible to tolerate. The psychoanalyst of that era did not medicate the psychoanalytic neurotic and was extremely reluctant to give drugs even to the dangerous, hospitalized paranoid schizophrenic. Drugs were slipped to the latter in a "don't ask, don't tell" manner.

In fact, 60 percent of the hospitalized patients were on tranquilizers or antidepressants, but no one made a great point of this embarrassing statistic to Dr. Semrad. I give you this bit of history so you can share my surprise when I read an article by Drs. Stephen Donovan and Steven Roose in the May 1995 issue of the *Journal of Clinical Psychiatry*. Donovan and Roose surveyed forty-five training analysts at the Columbia University Center for Psychoanalytic Training and Research and discovered that 18 percent of 277 patients in analysis were on a psychiatric drug, that most of them were depressed and on an SSRI, and that both the patient's mood and the analytic process improved. They noted that this contradicts "the belief that medication undermines the psychoanalytic situation." If Dr. Semrad is watching from heaven, he just learned something. But there are still psychotherapists of the old school who resist the idea of their clients and patients taking SSRIs or other psychoactive drugs. If you are currently seeing a physician like this, I suggest you tactfully urge a psychopharmacological consult. If the SSRI-resister is your family doctor and he or she lectures you about willpower, but willpower repeatedly fails you so that you cannot get yourself to do the things you know you need to do—such as talk to your children, perform with more energy at work, be nice to your spouse, or call your friends—then I suggest you tell your family practitioner you want to see a psychiatrist for evaluation and possible SSRI treatment, and that willpower may work for him or her, but you are sick and need treatment.

Is It Safe to Switch from Prozac to Paxil Without Waiting Two Weeks in Between?

Margaret Kreider, Ph.D., of SmithKline Beecham Pharmaceuticals, et al. studied the switch from Prozac to Paxil in two groups of over one hundred patients each, one of which was switched from Prozac to Paxil immediately, and the other of which had two weeks of a placebo in between. They found that the switch was equally well tolerated by both groups (*Journal of Clinical Psychiatry*, April 1995). Since Prozac remains in the blood for several weeks after its use is discontinued, many people are concerned about switching from Prozac to Paxil without waiting at least two weeks. As I have noted before, over 40 percent of depressed patients do not get better on the first drug given, either because of an inability to tolerate the side effects or because the drug fails to work. Therefore, questions of when and how to switch to another antidepressant are not academic but of practical, clinical importance. The changeovers must be considered carefully since some are dangerous and require a washout period in which no drug is given. The switch from Prozac to Paxil is not one of these.

Discontinuing Use of SSRIs

Since Prozac is a long-acting drug that remains in the blood for weeks, the changeover from it to Paxil is tolerated, even though it is sudden. Nonetheless, discontinuing use of SSRIs is best done gradually in order to spare patients unnecessary upset. I have observed what Dr. James Ellison calls a "withdrawal buzz," a painful "shock" in the head (also described as a "jolt" or "rush") in people who suddenly stop taking an SSRI. Why this occurs is unknown, but what is known is that it is not dangerous to the brain, and patients do not faint because of it. It is unpleasant, though, and can be avoided by very gradually tapering off use of the drug. Sometimes, as in the event of a severe allergic reaction to the drug, there is no choice, and use of the SSRI must be stopped suddenly. Any ill effects can be handled by an unrelated medication, but often there is no need.

Social Phobia and the SSRIs

The *Diagnostic and Statistical Manual of Mental Disorders* (4th ed., 1994) of the American Psychiatric Association defines social phobia as a "marked and persistent fear of one or more social or performance situations in which the person is exposed to unfamiliar people or to possible scrutiny by others." The person is in fear of humiliating or embarrassing himself, and either avoids such situations or endures them with anxiety. There is a movement among researchers and patients suffering from the condition to change the name to social anxiety disorder because social anxiety, with its attendant physical symptoms, underlies the secondary phobic avoidance behavior. Those who endure the stressful situation can be said to have social anxiety without phobic avoidance. Others, whose condition is lifelong and severe, can be diagnosed as having an avoidant personality disorder. The avoidance and intense anxiety interferes with the person's work, school, and/or social life. The condition can either be generalized, as in extreme shyness and avoidance, or be confined to one area, such as public speaking.

Considering that it is estimated that 20 million Americans will become social phobics sometime in their lifetime, and that this would make it the third most common psychiatric condition after major depression episodes and alcohol dependence, remarkably little is known about it. Twice as many women as men have it, often since early adolescence. In fact, 80 percent of cases occur before age twenty-five, and because it is chronic, it severely interferes with the person's life, since they avoid speaking in front of groups or to strangers, meeting new people, or eating in public. As a result, according to Dr. Lewis Judd, two thirds of social phobics are unmarried, half never completed high school, and 20 percent are unable to work. Unlike agoraphobics, who avoid places for fear of having a panic attack, social phobics avoid situations where they may be evaluated, ridiculed, or humiliated.

It is believed, based on studies, that genetic factors play an important role.

An article by Dr. Randall Marshall in the *Journal of Clinical Psychiatry* (June 1994) quotes two figures for the odds of suffering social phobia within one's lifetime: 2.4 percent and 13.3 percent. One figure is more than five times the other. No wonder efforts to find biological markers for the condition have been unsuccessful. Clearly, it is poorly defined. Jerome Kagan, who has studied shyness, describes a severe type of social phobia resulting in rapid pulse and overwhelming anxiety when a child is separated from its mother and confronted with new situations. But Dr. Kagan also describes a more moderate type of social phobia, one that can be overcome at a cocktail party filled with strangers by the simple downing of a first drink.

In spite of the lack of solid, scientific, objective criteria acceptable to all authorities as the cause and basis for cure of social phobia, I have seen this condition repeatedly during my psychiatric career, and watched it destroy many people's lives. The woman who is lonely and wants to meet men, but cannot bring herself to meet people who may judge and/or ridicule her, continues to sit at home alone. The graduate student who is terrified every time he goes to class that the professor might call on him. The consultant who cannot sleep the night before he makes a presentation before a client and becomes tongue-tied and does badly. The member of the symphony orchestra who shakes so badly she cannot play. The student who cannot give his oral report or who freezes during an examination. Social phobia is a real condition, a terrible condition, and one that ruins lives, but it is also a mild condition, something we all feel to some extent in the presence of strangers, in front of audiences, when we are going to be judged. At worst, it is a terrible affliction that can ruin lives. At best, it can be a source of mild social discomfort. If you think you have social phobia and have been losing out on your life, you should consult a psychotherapist and consider taking one of the following drugs:

B-adrenergic blockers
   propranolol (Inderal)
   atenolol (Tenormin)
   nadolol (Corgard)
Monoamine oxidase inhibitors
   phenelzine (Nardil)
   tranylcypromine (Parnate)
Benzodiazepines
   clonazepam (Klonopin)
   alprazolam (Xanax)
SSRIs—Prozac, Zoloft, Paxil, Luvox, Celexa, Lexapro
Buspirone (Buspar)

Inderal is the well-known stage-fright drug that stops the motor manifestations of anxiety such as hand-shaking, sweating, and racing pulse. It is taken by musicians and actors. It is sometimes handed out without a prescription by theater directors, which is not a good idea, since it should not be taken by asthmatics and can dangerously lower the blood pressure. Clearly, a doctor's supervision is called for. Inderal should be taken twenty to thirty minutes before a performance, such as public speaking, playing a stringed instrument, or exercising a skill in public that requires a steady hand. Tenormin and Corgard, which are prescribed less often, work similarly to Inderal. In generalized social phobia, which occurs in all social situations, as opposed to only a few circumstances, B-blockers are of no use.

The MAOIs (monoamine oxidase inhibitors) Nardil and Parnate are effective in the treatment of generalized social phobias, decreasing a person's excessive sensitivity to being viewed and judged. The problem with the MAOIs is their side effects and the dietary restrictions necessitated by their use. It is hoped that the much less problematic SSRIs (to be described next) will be equally effective in treating generalized social phobics, but controlled studies remain to be done. In the office and anecdotally, the SSRIs seem fine.

Buspirone, an antianxiety agent with serotonin effects, may

also be of some use, but there is considerable doubt about its efficacy in social phobia.

The antianxiety agents Xanax and Klonopin are of help in treating generalized social phobia, as are behavior and cognitive therapies.

The SSRIs (Prozac, Zoloft, Paxil, Luvox, and Celexa) have all been used to treat social phobia. They have been found effective in the studies done, but many of these have been open, as opposed to double-blind placebo-controlled, which means they are flawed because both the researcher and the patient knew that an SSRI was being given, and their expectations may have colored the results. In May 1999, Paxil became the first drug approved by the FDA for the treatment of social anxiety disorder (also called social phobia). In a twelve-week double-blind study of 183 patients, 55 percent of those on Paxil were much improved compared to 24 percent on a placebo. Patients may do better on 40 mg than on 20 mg, and it seems to take several months before the full benefit is experienced. Other SSRIs will probably also be effective. It is not known whether Klonopin, a benzodiazepine, is more or less effective. Some have suggested combining the two when one does not work. Studies in children will soon be undertaken, since social anxiety can cause school avoidance and school phobia.

Once again, the borders of social phobia present a research and therapeutic problem. Not only is there the border between normal stranger anxiety and excessive fear, but there is the border with other psychiatric conditions. Most social phobics also have either panic disorder, simple phobia, or obsessive-compulsive disorder. Furthermore, many are depressed because of their narrow lives, lack of confidence, and perhaps because whatever it is that makes them avoid new people and situations also makes them depressed. High sensitivity to rejection exists in both social phobics and depressives. MAOIs and SSRIs reduce this interpersonal hypersensitivity, allowing the individual to care less about what others may think and thus to go out into the world.

Obsessive-Compulsive Disorder (OCD)

Obsessive-compulsive disorder is characterized by obsessions and compulsions that are usually chronic. Obsessions refer to recurrent and unwanted thoughts that cause anxiety and discomfort because of their aggressive, sexual, or disgusting content. They include such things as fear of dirt and harm to the self or others. OCD patients are plagued by doubt about whether their hands are clean or the door is locked. Compulsions are behaviors such as hand-washing and checking the stove or door lock. OCD is not to be confused with compulsive personality. The OCD patient suffers from a compulsion that must be resisted, whereas the obsessive-compulsive personality disorder patient is happy in his orderliness and stinginess. The former rarity and now commonness (a lifetime rate of 2.5 percent) of OCD is attributed to these patients' secretiveness about their symptoms. To determine if you have OCD, ask yourself whether you have repetitive thoughts that seem horrible or weird, or things you do over and over again.

A 1984 National Epidemiologic Catchment Area (ECA) survey found that OCD was fifty to one hundred times more common than previously believed, affecting 1 to 2 percent of the population worldwide, and making it the fourth most common psychiatric disorder (after phobias, substance abuse, and major depression). There are two problems with this finding. One is that lay interviewers were used, and second, even more importantly, no careful evaluation of how the symptoms impaired the OCD sufferers was made. However, other studies have addressed these shortcomings, and found OCD to be as common as the ECA survey showed. Patients with OCD are more likely to also have schizophrenia, depression, Tourette's syndrome (involuntary muscle tics and vocal tics including obscene words), and other anxiety disorders.

The SSRIs have become the primary treatment for OCD, along with the tricyclic clomipramine. Serotonin has been studied in OCD and is found to have a role, as it does in aggression, anxiety, learning, social dominance, impulsivity, and suicide. Clomipramine has a potent serotonin effect, and is more effective against OCD than is desipramine, which is a norepinephrine-specific tricyclic. All the SSRIs have proved effective in treating OCD and, combined with behavior therapy, offer those suffering from this painful and debilitating condition real hope of spending less time obsessing, checking, hoarding, and washing, and more time with family, friends, and in meaningful work. This combination therapy helps most people get a lot better, but does not cure them completely. Because OCD is a chronic illness that waxes and wanes, SSRI treatment must be long-term. Symptomatic improvement may continue steadily for months.

Panic Disorder and the SSRIs

Panic disorder is a condition consisting of recurrent, spontaneous attacks of intense fear accompanied by some or all of the following: palpitations, sweating, shaking, shortness of breath, a choking feeling, chest pain, nausea, dizziness, numbness, chills, hot flashes, and feelings of unreality, of going crazy, or of dying. Panic attacks can be caused by a specific or social phobia or by post-traumatic stress disorder (a flashback), or they can be unexpected. In panic disorder, patients suddenly and unexpectedly feel faint, their hearts pound, they fear they will die, and they have difficulty breathing. They are often young adults who have recently experienced one of the following: the death of a loved one, a life-threatening illness or accident, separation from their family, thyroid disease, the birth of a child, or the taking of a mind-altering drug. Many panic disorder patients had school phobia as children.

Tricyclic antidepressants have been repeatedly demonstrated in carefully conducted controlled trials to stop panic attacks in patients who are not depressed. Imipramine, a tricyclic antidepressant highly effective in treating panic disorder, is also used in children with school phobia, making them able to leave their mothers and go to school. Imipramine does not stop the patient's fear of the next attack. This so-called anticipatory anxiety may require a benzodiazepine such as Valium, Ativan, or Klonopin. MAOIs and other tricyclic antidepressants also block panic attacks.

The SSRIs are also very effective in the treatment of panic. Like Imipramine, Prozac can also overstimulate panic patients if started at the usual 20-mg dose. To avoid this, the drug is started at 5 mg a day and raised 5 mg every week until 20 mg is reached, which is usually enough. The panic attacks are usually controlled within four to twelve weeks. It is not known exactly how long someone will have to stay on antidepressant drug therapy to prevent recurrence of panic attacks. Since it is a chronic disorder that improves and relapses, the therapy may have to go on a long time.

The benzodiazepines Xanax and Klonopin have also proved effective in the treatment of panic. Studies are under way comparing them with the antidepressants. They have fewer initial side effects than antidepressants, act faster, and are also effective against fear of the next attack, but because of concerns, which I believe are unfounded, that they are addicting, their use is reserved until antidepressants fail. Most psychopharmacologists believe that the problem of addiction to benzodiazepines (Valium, Xanax, Ativan, etc.) has been exaggerated, and applies to addicts rather than the general population, which is able to stop taking them when they are no longer needed without serious consequences.

Side Effects of the SSRIs

Nausea without vomiting, loose stools and diarrhea, nervousness and anxiety, loss of appetite, insomnia, headache, and sexual dysfunction are all potential side effects of the SSRIs. As treatment continues, many of the side effects go away, especially nausea and headache. Some of the symptoms, such as anxiety, headache, loss of sex drive, and abdominal distress, are due to the depression itself, and not to the drug. In general, the higher the dose of the drug, the more side effects. It therefore makes sense to start at as low a dosage as possible and move up gradually. Antidepressants work slowly, taking days to weeks, and the tendency to increase the dosage instead of waiting for the therapeutic effect produces no added benefit and causes more side effects than are necessary. When side effects do occur, the dose can be reduced or divided or taken at a different time of day, another antidepressant can be tried, or the side effects can be treated.

Nausea

This can be a problem with any of the SSRIs, but if the drug is taken with food or the dose decreased, it is tolerable. After a few weeks, nausea disappears. About 25 percent of people on SSRIs become nauseous, but only 5 percent have to discontinue the drug because of it. It is now thought that the gastric agent Cisapride is too dangerous to use to combat antidepressant-induced nausea. Lower doses and more gradual increases lessen nausea.

Insomnia

All the SSRIs cause insomnia in about 20 percent of those who take them. This can be minimized by taking the drug in the morning and, if this fails, lessening the dose until the symptom disappears, in which case the dose can be raised again. Sometimes the insomnia is due not to the SSRI but to worsening depression, drug-caused muscle restlessness, or mania. If the insomnia continues, an additional sedating antidepressant can be prescribed, such as trazodone (Desyrel, etc.), or a benzodiazepine, such as triazolam (Halcion) flurazepam (Dalmane), or a non-benzodiazepine hypnotic, such as zaleplon (Sonata) or zolpidem (Ambien), at bedtime.

Nervousness and Anxiety

Especially at the beginning of treatment, about 20 percent of people feel "wired," jittery, restless, irritable, and shaky. It may be due to the SSRI, or to worsening depression, incipient mania, or drug-induced motor restlessness called akathisia, the inability to remain still, which is associated with bodily rocking and shifting from leg to leg occasionally occurring as a side effect of the SSRIs and Serzone, and which can be relieved by propranolol (Inderal and others) and/or a benzodiazepine such as Klonopin. If it is due to the SSRI, dose reduction and waiting to get used to the drug often works. Then the dose can be raised gradually. If the "wired" feeling continues, the drug can be changed to another antidepressant, or an antianxiety drug like Valium or Ativan be added.

Headache

Headache is a very common symptom of major depression. SSRIs may induce or exacerbate tension and migraine headaches. In fact, SSRIs cause more headaches than do the older tricyclic antidepressants. As with other side effects, alternative causes of headache must be considered and ruled out. The dosage can be reduced while the patient gets used to the drug; changes in diet, exercise, and stress reduction can be advised, aspirin taken as needed, or small doses of Elavil added.

Weight Gain

The SSRIs are certainly better than the older antidepressants regarding weight gain. Most people are able to undergo a full course of treatment without gaining a pound. Occasionally, a person on an SSRI will gain a lot of weight. This may be due to untreated depression, since some depressives overeat, and many are underactive. Sometimes weight gain is due to thyroid dysfunction.

I advise people on SSRIs to watch the scale regularly, to

exercise, and to seek nutritional counseling should their weight increase. Occasionally, the addition of the stimulants Dexedrine or Ritalin to the SSRI will increase the antidepressant effect and decrease weight. The overwhelming majority of the people I have treated do not end up abusing Dexedrine or Ritalin when it is used for this purpose, but many drugstores, because of governmental harassment and fear of break-ins, no longer stock Dexedrine.

Hypomania and Mania

Every antidepressant can be associated with mania, but whether the drug actually causes it or otherwise unearths it in individuals who would become manic anyway is an ongoing debate among experts. If you are taking an SSRI and you suddenly feel extraordinarily happy, your thoughts begin to race, you sleep only a couple of hours a night, you have boundless energy, you start to spend money you do not have, and you begin to engage in business activities and romantic liaisons that horrify your friends and family, then use of the antidepressant must be stopped immediately and the doctor called right away. If you have only a mild version and feel just a little speeded up and unable to sleep, a dosage reduction may be all you need.

If you know you are bipolar (manic-depressive) or have relatives who are, be sure to tell your doctor before starting an SSRI. But if you are an outpatient dysthymic or other depressive type who needs an SSRI, you probably have little reason to worry that it will suddenly make you manic.

Drowsiness

About 20 percent of people on SSRIs feel drugged or drowsy, and about 5 percent discontinue use of the drug because of it. Although less frequent than with the older tricyclics, it can still be a problem. Sometimes drowsiness is due to the SSRI-induced insomnia, but often not. If drowsiness occurs, it is best to take the drug in the evening, and if this fails, to lower the dose. Also, try an extra cup of coffee in the morning.

Sexual Dysfunction

Disturbances in sexual functioning have emerged as the principal problem with the SSRIs and have caused many people to stop taking them, often at the risk of becoming depressed again. Initially reported in the *Physicians' Desk Reference (PDR)* as a low occurrence rate, it is now estimated at 30 to 50 percent or higher. The reason it was initially missed is that there is no requirement that drug-induced sexual difficulties be a topic of questioning in prerelease drug trials. If not asked, people, particularly women, are not likely to mention them, especially when they are being treated for major depression.

The sexual difficulties caused by the SSRIs include: decrease or absence of sexual desire; delayed, painful, or absence of orgasm; and erectile dysfunction.

While it is necessary to remember that sexual problems are widespread in the general population, and that diminished desire is certainly common in the depressed (and is, in fact, one factor in its diagnosis), there is no question that SSRI-induced sexual difficulties are a major problem, causing people not to want to take the drug, and to stop taking it when they should continue.

Take the case of Barbara. She loved sex with her husband throughout the eighteen years of their marriage. While their relationship had otherwise been stormy as they struggled on limited funds to bring up their children, their bedroom was their salvation. Unfortunately, there was major depression in Barbara's family, and she, too, had had numerous episodes of it, never requiring hospitalization, but nonetheless quite debilitating. She would be confined to her bed for days at a time, get headaches, backaches, and stomach problems, and lose days at work. Fortunately, antidepressants had helped her over the years, but the tricyclics had made her gain weight, which she struggled in vain to lose. Barbara welcomed the SSRIs because of their reputation of not causing users to put on poundage. But they ruined her desire and her capacity for orgasm. As soon as she recovered from her latest episode of depression, she stopped taking them, even though she realized she had a good chance of getting depressed again. It was not long before this happened.

A growing list of ways to cope with the SSRI sexual side effect is largely anecdotal and may be effective. The simplest is dose reduction and waiting for the problem to go away, but this is far from always what happens. People taking Zoloft or Paxil (this does not work with long-acting Prozac) can skip the drug a day or two before anticipated sexual activity. The second is switching to Wellbutrin, Serzone, or Remeron, with continued antidepressant effect and normalization of sexual function. If these latter three antidepressants were as good as the SSRIs in every other way and had fewer or no sexual side effects, then the issue could easily be resolved by people taking them in the first place and skipping the SSRIs; but these drugs have other detriments (discussed in Chapter 4) so the SSRIs remain the first choice among most psychiatrists. But once the SSRI sexual side effect gets out of hand, this may be a sensible alternative. Short of stopping use of the SSRIs because of sexual side effects, a variety of drugs have been tried to reverse the problem. The reports of their success are anecdotal and not well studied. They include:

Bethanechol (Urecholine, etc.)

Taken thirty minutes to two hours before sexual activity, bethanechol has been shown to be effective in overcoming sexual dysfunction. It is not to be taken by patients with asthma, ulcers, or cardiac disease, and can worsen diarrhea induced by the SSRIs, as well as causing a running nose, excessive tearing, and stomach cramps. A similar drug (neostigmine) can also be used.

Yohimbine (Yocon, Yohimex, etc.)

Taken two to four hours before intercourse, yohimbine seems to correct all sexual problems, including lack of desire, arousal, orgasm, and ejaculation, but the studies have been open rather than double-blind controlled, and require verification. The dosage seems somewhat difficult to adjust since too little does no good, and too much makes people feel shaky, wired, anxious, or tense. Nonetheless, it seems to work pretty well, and I have tried it in a few patients with success. Other yohimbine side effects include nausea, increased heart rate, blood pressure, and irritability, but they are usually not serious. While the *PDR* may be overly cautious in warning against its use in females or in psychiatric patients, my experience has been that it works well in both. The *PDR* further warns that the drug should not be used with antidepressants, which may be true for the tricyclics, but not for the SSRIs. The *PDR* warns against the use of yohimbine in pregnant women and anyone suffering from renal disease or gastric ulcers.

Cyproheptadine (Periactin, etc.)

Cyproheptadine is an antiserotonin antihistamine that has been used to reverse SSRI sexual dysfunction. I have resisted using it because it can reverse the antidepressant effect of the SSRIs. Drugs that raise the level of serotonin in the brain lower the sex drive.

Dopamine

The neurotransmitter dopamine has been shown to increase male sexual behavior in rats, and drugs that increase the level of dopamine have been observed to increase penile erection. It has been reported that Parkinson's patients on levodopa, a drug converted to dopamine in the body and used to treat parkinsonism, have increased libido, spontaneous erections, and nocturnal emissions. Because of these reports, several dopamine-raising drugs have been tried to relieve SSRI-induced sexual dysfunction. They are:

Amantadine
Dextroamphetamine
Pemoline (Cylert)—pemoline can cause liver damage and
should be avoided for this purpose.
Bromocriptine (Parlodel)

Wellbutrin

Wellbutrin can be added in an attempt to reverse any sexual
inhibition caused by ongoing SSRI treatment. Unfortunately,
it is not very effective in doing so. When taken alone, Wellbutrin usually does not adversely affect sexual functioning.
Serzone and Remeron are also less likely to adversely affect
sexual functioning, but are not added to reverse sexual dysfunction as is Wellbutrin.

Viagra

Viagra (sildenafil) has been found to increase orgasm ability
and sexual desire in men and women on SSRIs. At doses of 50
to 100 mg per day, it is more effective in men than in women.
It should not be used by anyone taking nitroglycerin or a similar drug for angina, because a sharp blood-pressure drop might
occur, resulting in a heart attack. Common Viagra side effects
are headache, visual disturbances, flushing, and nasal conges-
tion. The dose is 50 mg one hour before sex, and the maximum
dose is 100 mg. Sometimes a half pill, 25 mg, is enough.

Serotonin Syndrome (SS)

When an SSRI and an MAOI (Nardil, Parnate, etc.) are
administered together or within two to five weeks of each
other, the serotonin syndrome (SS) can occur. Characterized
by fever, sweating, rapid pulse, high blood pressure, rigidity,
confusion, and disturbed consciousness, it can result in coma
or death. Patients with Parkinson's disease often become
depressed and are treated with an antidepressant. If they are
on Eldepryl, an MAOI used to treat Parkinson's, giving them
an SSRI can occasionally be dangerous and produce the sero-

tonin syndrome. Ultram, a new drug for pain relief, when combined with an SSRI can also cause the serotonin syndrome, as can Demerol. Imitrex, the serotonin drug used in patients with migraine headaches, may possibly interact with SSRIs, but this danger has not been firmly established. Zomig, like Imitrex a drug for migraine, must also be used carefully when combined with an SSRI. Unless mixed with another serotonin-elevating drug, the SSRIs do not cause SS, and are safe.

Sweating and Dry Mouth

Sweating and dry mouth are not common problems with the SSRIs, but they do occur. Dry mouth can be combated with sugar-free gum and candies and drops of artificial saliva. Dental caries should be guarded against by careful mouth hygiene.

Some increase in sweating, especially in the upper body, may occur during SSRI treatment. If it becomes very heavy, it may be a sign of fever. Use of the drug should be stopped, and your doctor called.

Hair Loss

Hair loss can occur with tricyclic antidepressants, the SSRIs, and Serzone. While it happens with one antidepressant, it may not with another. This side effect is not common but occurs more often in women.

Bleeding

SSRIs and Effexor may affect clotting by their effect on serotonin and thus on platelets. Bruising or bleeding are sometimes due to serotonergic antidepressants.

Antidepressants During Pregnancy and Lactation

When possible, depressed pregnant women should be treated by psychotherapy alone. The studies of newborns whose mothers were treated with SSRIs have not revealed any gross abnormalities, and if medication is necessary to prevent depression, it is safer to continue an SSRI throughout pregnancy than to stop it. A mother's untreated depression can harm the development of language, thinking, and behavior in her infant and children. If breast feeding is done while a woman takes an antidepressant, infants are exposed to very small amounts, and most do not seem to be harmed, although occasionally an infant may build up high levels of the drug. Babies must be carefully monitored by a doctor if the mother took a drug during pregnancy or continues to do so while nursing. The amount of drug in breast milk is small, and to date, no significant adverse effects have been discovered.

Tolerating the SSRIs

Nearly every textbook and journal article says that Paxil and the other SSRIs are well tolerated, and therefore ideal for months and years of maintenance therapy to prevent recurrence. I believe it would be more accurate to say the SSRIs are better tolerated than the older tricyclics. Eugene Duboff, M.D., in his article entitled "Long-Term Treatment of Major Depressive Disorder with Paroxetine [Paxil]" in the December 1993 *Journal of Clinical Psychopharmacology*, records that during a one-year trial on Paxil, "adverse events caused approximately 30 percent of patients to withdraw from the study prematurely." The most common reasons cited were fatigue or sleepiness, nausea, headaches, and sweatiness. He goes on to assert that the drug was well tolerated. This does not sound like "well tolerated" to me. In an eight-week double-blind placebo- and Elavil-controlled study of Zoloft in outpatients with major depression by Frederick W. Reimherr et al., reported in the December 1990 *Journal of Clinical Psychiatry*, the dropout rate in all three patient groups was the same, although the reasons cited were different. In the placebo groups, lack of efficacy was the main cause, while in the drug groups, it was side effects (about 20 percent for Elavil and Zoloft). The Zoloft patients had gastrointestinal complaints and sexual dysfunctions, while the Elavil group suffered from more sleepiness and fatigue, constipation, blurred vision, trouble urinating, and dizziness. Although the dropout rate was the same, the Elavil patients had more and worse side effects. In another eight-week double-blind study comparing Zoloft and Elavil in elderly depressed patients, Cal K. Cohn, M.D., et al., reported (also in the December 1990 *Journal of Clinical Psychiatry*) a dropout rate of 28 percent for Zoloft and 35 percent for Elavil. Zoloft won, but hardly overwhelmingly. Without quoting all the other studies and statistics, which make for dull reading, I only wish to sum up by saying that the SSRIs are better tolerated in most studies than Elavil and Tofranil, but their side effects still cause about 20 percent of those taking them to drop out within six weeks, and probably another 10 percent within the first year. There are real advantages to the SSRIs, which I will summarize at the end of this chapter, but they are not perfect, and many people have difficulty tolerating them.

Drug/SSRI Interactions

Since you may be on an SSRI for months, even years, it is important to know how other drugs that you may be taking, or may need to take in the future, will be affected by the SSRIs. Fortunately, the list of serious interactions is not long. Since the SSRIs are metabolized by the liver, they may force up the blood level of a second drug broken down in the same way. If the second drug has a narrow margin between its therapeutic action and toxic level, this can be dangerous. Another source of interaction trouble occurs when two drugs act on the same target. Thus, SSRIs can increase the tremors caused by lithium, and can also produce the serotonin syndrome when combined with MAOIs (which should never be done) and, to a lesser extent, with tryptophan and meperidine (Demerol). This interaction can be especially dangerous when an MAOI is given within six weeks after use of Prozac has been discontinued, since it takes that long for Prozac to be completely cleared from the body. Effexor, Serzone, Remeron, Anafranil, and Ultram (a pain medication) can also cause the serotonin syndrome when combined with an MAOI. Combining Paxil and Desyrel can also cause the serotonin syndrome.

When tricyclics are combined with SSRIs (in cases where the SSRIs alone are not successful), it must be remembered that less than the normal dose of the tricyclic should be taken, because the SSRI forces the blood level of the tricyclic up two or more times, which could be dangerous if the normal dose were used.

When beginning SSRI treatment, some people become sleepy, and will become more so if they drink alcohol. But those who are not made sleepy by SSRIs can drink their normal amount without any added effect from the drug.

Only MAOIs and tryptophan must be avoided with the SSRIs. The drugs listed below must be used cautiously because of interactions, and under the close supervision of your physician.

Drugs Interacting with All SSRIs
Anticonvulsants
Lithium
Antiarrhythmics
Beta-blockers
Anticoagulants
Antihistamines
Antiulcer drugs
Antianxiety drugs
Phenothiazine antipsychotics
Tricyclic antidepressants

The antidepressants least likely to cause interactions are Effexor, Celexa, and Lexapro, making them commonly used in older patients likely to be on other medical drugs.

SSRI Dosage

Dosage depends on the individual patient and must be set after careful consultation between you and your physician. In general, if your symptoms are not unbearable, it makes sense to start low and increase the dosage slowly. The following table can be used as a guide.

	Starting Dose (mg)	Tablet/Capsule Sizes (mg)	Daily Dose (mg)
Prozac (fluoxetine)	5–20	10, 20	20–80
Zoloft (sertraline)	25–50	25, 50, 100	50–200
Paxil (paroxetine)	10–20	10, 20, 30, 40	20–50
Luvox (fluvoxamine)	50	25, 50, 100	150–300
Celexa (citalopram)	20	20, 40	20–40
Lexapro (escitalopram)	10	10, 20	10–20

Some people can tolerate 20 mg of Prozac from the start, but many feel wired or drugged, or suffer abdominal distress, and do better on 5 or 10 mg. The manufacturer (Eli Lilly) later issued a 10-mg capsule and most recently a 10-mg scored tablet easily divided in half, because many people could not take 20 mg right away. Lilly also came out with a liquid form containing 20 mg per teaspoon for those who wish to find out exactly how much they need. From a financial point of view, the 20-mg capsule is cheapest, and the liquid form most expensive. Two 10-mg capsules cost much more than one 20-mg capsule. It may be wise to get a small supply of 10s at first and, once you are comfortable on 20 mg, to shift over. Zoloft comes in scored tablets of 50 and 100 mg, so that it can be divided in half (or less), and Paxil comes in 10-, 20- (scored), 30-, and 40-mg tablets. Luvox comes in 25- (unscored) and in 50- and

100-mg scored tablets. Celexa comes in 20- and 40-mg scored tablets. Lexapro comes in 10- and 20-mg scored tablets.

The rate of dosage elevation should be slowest for Prozac, since it builds up in the body over several weeks. For those starting on 20 mg, no increase should be attempted within the first month, even if there has been little response. Then 10 mg more per month might be tried. Those who are impatient and want to hurry the elevation may pay the price of more side effects, but these are almost always annoying rather than serious, and for those people in a lot of distress, it may be worth it. Prozac is best taken in the morning with food, unless it causes drowsiness, in which case it should be taken after the evening meal.

Zoloft can be taken after the evening meal, as can Paxil, unless it causes agitation or insomnia, in which case it can be taken after breakfast. It can be started with a whole pill or half of one pill, and moved up every week or two until a full response occurs. If after a maximum of several months of 200 mg of Zoloft or 50 mg of Paxil there is still no response, use of the drug should be discontinued. Use of the SSRIs should not be discontinued suddenly, but slowly and gradually.

Luvox can be begun at 50 mg and increased to a maximum of 300 mg. It has been released in the United States only for obsessive compulsive disorder, but has been used worldwide for depression with success.

Much has been made of the fact that Prozac is eliminated from the body only gradually, and some argue that the side effects last much longer because of this. For this reason, many believe that shorter-acting Paxil and Zoloft are more desirable. In my practice, I have not found it to make much difference. If the next drug planned is an MAOI after an SSRI failure, then the wait would only have to be two weeks with Paxil and Zoloft instead of five weeks with Prozac, but that is a theoretical advantage which only rarely comes up.

What's in a Name?

The naming of modern antidepressants is no accident. Clearly, I do not know what went on behind closed doors as the pharmaceutical companies went over what to call these wonder drugs, but here are some of my associations to how they are trying to subliminally influence doctors to prescribe and patients to take these agents.

Prozac. What would have happened if it had been called antizac?

Zoloft. *Zo* refers to the Greek *zoe*, or life, and *loft*, to propel in a high arc.

Paxil. From the Latin word *pax*, which means peace, the opposite of anguish.

Wellbutrin. To be well, not ill.

Effexor. To be effective and competent. Latin *efficere*, to accomplish.

Serzone. Calm, as in serene.

Luvox. In Latin, *vox* means voice, but this name is not satisfactory unless one knows that *luv* means love in old English.

Remeron. A *remedy* for depression, or REMeron to restore normal REM sleep.

Celexa. A highly *selective* SSRI.

Lexapro. A left-handed professional.

In the following section, I will provide detailed explorations of Prozac, Zoloft, Paxil, Luvox, Celexa, and Lexapro.

Prozac (Fluoxetine)

Now Generic

No longer protected by patent, Prozac is now available as generic fluoxetine. Third-party payers encourage the generic, and discourage, with various penalties, the brand.

The generic versus brand controversy has occasioned a fair

degree of debate over the years, no matter what the drug involved. The brand side usually says the two are not clinically equivalent, but are absorbed differently and the effect compromised. They also say the generic ingredients are inferior, and at times are gotten from unhygienic Third World sources. Governmental inspection of their manufacture is incomplete. The small number of large pharmaceutical companies manufacturing the brand products are much easier to police than the scores of little operations turning out the generics. What could be substantial savings for the consumer are often gobbled up by greedy retail pharmacies, who mark the generics down 30 percent from the brands when they could be 90 percent cheaper. The third-party payers have considerably more clout than the individual consumer, but nonetheless allow the drugstore to make a much larger profit on the generic than they ought.

Should you insist on the brand if you have been on it for years? I would, while fully aware that my insistence is probably more emotional than rational. Would I be willing to submit a larger co-pay, demanded by my insurance company, than for the generic? I would. Would I be willing to pay the full sixty dollars or more monthly without any insurance contribution at all? Perhaps not.

Making the Prozac Decision

As Prozac has become overwhelmingly popular, the matter of who should take it has become muddled. Originally released for the treatment of major depression, its use has spread to many other conditions. Not only are people with eating, sexual, and anxiety disorders, depressives, schizophrenics, obsessive-compulsives, and posttraumatic stress disorder patients candidates for Prozac, but also those who are subsyndromal: the timid; those with low energy and low self-esteem; those who are irritable, perfectionist, inflexible, or suffering from a general malaise or unhappiness; and those who are too aggressive or abusive. In short, anyone—sick or not—may benefit from the civilizing effects of Prozac.

The physician legally controls distribution of the drug through the prescription pad, but since the definition of need (the so-called indication) is broad (one could say nonexistent), the patient's suffering and wish for the drug often become the deciding factors. Unfortunately, the nature of serotonin is about as clear as that of the id, and its effect on practice may be the same: everyone, no matter what the diagnosis, became a candidate for psychoanalysis or therapy, and now becomes one for Prozac. Twelve million Americans have taken Prozac. Much of this use is warranted, but clearly some is not. Except in cases of severe major depression, there is no science to guide the physician in the decision to prescribe Prozac. If there is marked interference with your daily functioning, and you are in a lot of pain, then you should persuade your doctor to let you try it for at least several months. The risk of harm is small, and the chance of benefit great.

The Benefits of Prozac

Large, controlled studies of Prozac have established its effectiveness in major depression to be equal to that of the tricyclic antidepressants (e.g., Elavil and Tofranil), with fewer side effects. There are studies of its use in other well-defined conditions which support its prescription in obsessive-compulsive disorder, bulimia, premenstrual dysphoric disorder, and other diagnostic types discussed in the earlier part of this chapter concerning SSRIs in general. With respect to its use in the timid, irritable, overly sensitive, insecure, and fatigued, and those lacking self-confidence, Prozac's success has been established by anecdote rather than controlled study. Anecdotal evidence can be as reliable as the reports of miracles, but that does not make either of them untrue. There are many people who believe Prozac has restored them to full functioning, and I am convinced from my own observation that they are right in their belief. But a large group feel only somewhat better, and others have been hurt by the drug. It is the physician's duty to know what can go wrong and watch for it carefully over time, even if the decision to take Prozac has been handed over to the patient out of the doctor's ignorance, as opposed to carelessness. If a person says to me that he is suffering and I think there is a reasonable chance Prozac will relieve him, I feel obliged to prescribe it. I consider this no more irresponsible than if a postsurgical patient complained of pain and I issued a narcotic. However, I would not prescribe morphine for someone with chronic low-grade back pain, because it is dangerous to do so. The question is, how dangerous is it to prescribe Prozac for more vague, nondisease conditions, ones that are either subsyndromal or perhaps matters of temperament and character rather than syndromes or even subsyndromes?

How Does Prozac Work?

Because the serotonin story remains a mystery, and because no one has proven that depressives have too little of it, it seems more useful to think of Prozac's actions in terms used by those who take it.

In major depression, the reduction in anxiety, bodily aches and pains, trouble thinking and concentrating, sleep disturbance, motor retardation, and depressed mood has been measured both on the basis of patients' and physicians' accounts of their overall impressions and by means of specialized depression scales administered by trained raters who did not know if the patient was on a drug or a placebo. The way Prozac works in the large variety of other psychiatric disorders it has been used to treat is, I think, as follows:

As an Anti-Rage Drug

On Prozac, the physically abusive strike out less or not at all, the formerly irritable no longer scream in frustration, and the overly aggressive become less abrasive. Prozac can be thought of as a calming and civilizing drug.

The obvious bad side effect of this is that one can become

tranquil in situations in which it would be more appropriate
to cry out. One of my patients entered into an abusive intimate relationship while on Prozac. When he went off the
drug, he realized the relationship had been a terrible mistake. The doctor and the person considering Prozac must not
only identify the presence of anger, rage, and aggression, but
evaluate these emotions in the context of the person's life.
Are they signals that should be attended to and used as data
upon which to form judgments, or are they pathologic aber-
rations requiring Prozac for their removal?

Improved Effectiveness

Whether the source of feeling strong and in control comes
from the mind actually working better or from improved
morale and self-esteem, which bring the expectation of success, the person on Prozac has a sense of being more effective
and therefore likely to overcome obstacles. Thus, the person
with a history of social phobia is able to give a speech or enter
a room of strangers, and someone who never spoke up at
sales meetings will begin to do so.

The relationship of anxiety and depression to self-esteem
is well known. If your heart is racing with fear and dread of
the future, or if you feel stupid and inept because of depression, then you will not expect to overcome the novel and difficult situations you encounter at work or in your social life.
Whether your mind functions better, your self-esteem is
improved, your anxiety or depression relieved, or your hopes
raised—whatever the reason—you feel more in control and
effective, and thus your performance improves.

The Pleasure Center Is Turned On

Prozac is not a euphoriant giving people a high like marijuana or cocaine, but like other antidepressants, it turns on
the pleasure center that depression extinguishes. A main
reason why people feel depressed, lose interest in previously
enjoyed activities, stop eating, have no energy, and are unable
to concentrate and make decisions is that they anticipate

no pleasure from these activities. When Prozac activates the pleasure center, normal appetites and interests return. The depressive's social withdrawal ends; friends are called in the anticipation of a good time. Desire for food and sex returns because they promise enjoyment, and life seems worth sustaining. The pain and misery gone, pleasure once again rewards and motivates activities.

Decreased Sensitivity

Many depressives are thin-skinned and easily hurt by a snub or an unintended slight. They may agonize for hours after a social gathering about why someone did not speak to or dance with them or what a particular remark meant that seemed to wound them. Some of these sufferers actively seek one social event after another, motivated by a feeling of emptiness and sadness and a desire for relief through human contact, but often they are disappointed by snubs and rejections that less sensitive people would not even have noticed. Like many symptoms of depression, this one is connected to many of the others. If you feel worthless and have low self-esteem, you are much more easily hurt than if you are sure of yourself. If your pleasure center is turned off and you are already in pain, a snub hurts more than if you feel well. The same goes for criticism, which shakes the fragile equilibrium of the depressive, and therefore can be tolerated less well than by the nondepressed.

Prozac makes the depressed person less sensitive to slights and criticism, and more able to consider the suggestions of a boss or family member without overreacting with hurt or rage.

Increased Hope

Depressed people are negative about their abilities, and about the past and the future. Feeling without hope, they are unable to plan their lives, from the smallest social event to the largest project, and are plagued by passivity and indecision. If you ask them to the movies on a Saturday night, they cannot give a straight answer, since they do not know whether they will feel well enough to go. Once again, the symptoms of depression are related to one another. Without the ability to experience pleasure, it is hard to hope that future action will be fruitful. If you feel ineffective and worthless, it is impossible to believe that your efforts will be rewarded, so that you are filled with hopeful anticipation. Without hope, people sit still and alone, unable to motivate themselves to act. Once Prozac restores hope, the person begins to plan social activities, and at work is able to take the many small steps leading to the completion of a big project or sale.

What Is Unique About How Prozac Works?

The five things I have just discussed—decreased rage, increased self-esteem, activation of the pleasure center, diminished sensitivity, and the restoration of hope—are not unique to Prozac. The other SSRIs are all equally capable of producing these results. The older antidepressants certainly could turn on the pleasure center, restore hope, and increase self-esteem, but because of their tricky dose schedules (from one to twelve pills) and their annoying side effects (dry mouth, constipation, blood pressure drop, racing pulse, weight gain, blurred vision), their use was reserved for more severe depressions, and given in ineffective, inadequate dosages by nonspecialists. Thus, the large group of nonmajor depressives—the shy, the overly sensitive, the obsessed, the impulsive, the insecure, the irritable, and the aggressive—were rarely if ever medicated using the older antidepressants, and almost never in adequate dosages because the side effects would have made them intolerable.

In the general population, rage, along with physical and verbal abuse, nasty impatience, and a hostile confrontational attitude, are diminished by the SSRIs, as they never were before by the older antidepressants. Hypersensitivity to rejection and criticism, fearfulness, timidity, shyness, rigidity, perfectionism, and impulsivity are all affected by Prozac and the other SSRIs.

Prozac is not different from the other SSRIs, it was simply there first, used most, and has been the focus of the largest mythology. Zoloft, Paxil, Luvox, Celexa, and Lexapro have never appeared on the covers of popular magazines, or been singled out for attack by the Scientologists. Prozac is the name everybody knows, the one appearing on book titles. It is the drug people were likely to ask for. Now that generic fluoxetine is no longer advertised, those in pain are more likely to ask for the latest, such as Lexapro or Cymbalta, in the hope that they will be even more effective and less toxic.

Prozac Is an Old Drug

New drugs are like new lovers. First, there is the excitement of finding out about the promise of unknown benefits, accompanied by nervousness about undiscovered dangers. After a while, the pluses and minuses surface, resulting in a comfortable status quo or the decision to move on to someone or something better. Among the SSRIs and other newly available antidepressants, no one drug stands out as the best. They offer seductive alternatives, especially to those disappointed by Prozac. The attractions of the other antidepressants will be described in the sections in which they are considered, but some of these are siren songs with known and hidden dangers. Where possible, the use of older drugs whose characteristics are understood is safer and preferable to use of the latest one, whose harms are unknown.

Women and Prozac

As I begin to tell you about seven of the hundreds of people I have significantly helped with Prozac, I notice that five are women—slightly over 70 percent. Since most studies find that women make up 67 percent of those suffering from depressions, my 70 percent could simply reflect the national average. But many of the people I am about to describe are not major depressives. Rather, the fact that there is a preponderance of women reflects something else I have found in my clinical practice. Women are more willing to accept help when they need it, and do not have to be in the driver's seat or hold the TV remote control. Taking a psychiatric drug for depression or other mental condition is perceived by most people to be different from talking therapy, and to imply that the condition is more serious, that they cannot handle it by themselves and need medication. Many men resist this need, seeing it as a sign of weakness and a form of dependence. Women, perhaps more realistic and practical, are more willing to accept the necessary and to be open to advice from an expert. Men find it more threatening when they are ill and needy, subject to forces they cannot completely control. Since all human beings are subject to illness and forces beyond their control, perhaps men are the weaker sex in light of their reluctance to recognize and accept this state of nature.

Seven Prozac Success Stories

Although I am about to briefly tell you about seven Prozac successes, I must remind you that Prozac helps only about 30 percent of the severely depressed, and about 70 percent of all the depressed. It has done a lot of good, and continues to do so, but it is not a miracle drug. I include seven successes simply to show what it does when it works.

Out of Bed
Thirty-two-year-old Barbara needed to feel up and confident to go out on sales calls. Instead, she languished in bed and was in no condition to sell herself or her products. After two months of Prozac, she was not only back selling successfully but making plans for her future.

Tears and No Man
A thirty-six-year-old stranger in a new city, Laura burst into tears at work, and felt lonely, less capable than the other middle managers, and unable to attract a suitable man. Prozac steadily

raised her level of confidence and stopped her tears. Feeling better for six months, she decided to stop taking the drug, but her improvement continued. Performing well at work, she was promoted. She fell in love and has plans to marry.

No Longer Punching His Wife

Twenty-seven-year-old Jim would periodically punch and hurt his wife, but never touched the children. He denied being depressed or even angry with his wife, and said the blows (he sometimes hurt his fist punching the wall) were delivered impulsively, unexpectedly, and without reason. I made the diagnosis of intermittent explosive disorder and prescribed Prozac. The punches stopped.

The Ability and Courage to Speak Out

At the age of twenty-six, Eliza had just gotten a promotion that required her to make presentations to the senior management of her company, a prospect which terrified her: she was certain she would do badly. In addition, she was reluctant to speak up in other situations, even among her friends, because she believed her thoughts to be dull. She had long periods of social withdrawal accompanied by feelings of boredom, sadness, and low self-esteem. I made the diagnosis of dysthymia and started her on Prozac. Several weeks later, she felt vastly improved. Not only did she have the courage to speak up at senior management meetings, she was convinced her mind worked better.

Eliza not only felt more confident, her mind actually began to function better. One important factor in depression is its effect on thinking. The minds of depressed people are slowed; they experience a poverty of thoughts, their concentration is faulty, and in elderly people, depression can produce a false dementia with disorientation and impaired memory, judgment, and intellect. Eliza is not a dramatic person whose speech is filled with exaggeration. When she said her thoughts were more lucid, evolved, and complete when she was on Prozac, I tended to believe her.

Less Angry and Critical

Frank was fifty-five years old, worked hard as a college administrator, and came home tired and intolerant. He expected his wife to wait on him and to attend to the home, which was his oasis. She worked hard at her job, too, and wished to retire from her post as Frank's servant. Her failure to care for him properly enraged Frank, who looked daggers at her but said little. Instead, he poured himself a few too many stiff drinks, and sometimes these disinhibited him, and out poured vicious remarks toward his wife. These she attributed to the effects of alcohol rather than to the need for adjustments and compromises in their marriage. The diagnosis in this case was episodic alcoholism and marital relational problems. After several weeks on Prozac, Frank felt less inclined to drink and appeared less angry toward his wife. The angry look on his face had mostly disappeared.

Frank's case was not a Prozac cure. He continued to drink occasionally and to feel angry toward his wife. The value of the drug lay in the fact that he was more able to articulate his displeasure instead of silently raging or intermittently exploding aided by alcohol. The work with his psychotherapist was aided, not superseded, by the drug.

I'll Never Have a Family

Barbara was thirty-five, unmarried, anxious, and depressed that she would never have a family. Her superior intelligence, good looks, and attractive personality made her a success at work, but she remained miserable about her personal life, and was in therapy for several years with little success. Diagnostically, she was either a dysthymic (chronic mild depression) with an obsession about marriage and children, or a person with an obsessive-compulsive disorder who could not stop thinking about having a family; or perhaps she suffered from a mixed anxiety and depressive syndrome, and felt hopeless and worried about the future. Prozac brought her complete relief, no matter what the correct diagnosis. Those who see the drug as balancing the serotonin system do not worry so much about diagnostic distinctions. She ceased to be convinced of her inability to get what she wanted, and less obsessed, frantic, and depressed, she relaxed and started to achieve her goals. She found a man she loved and felt comfortable with, and began to hope that everything would work out and they would marry.

My Husband Is a Complete Egotist

Evelyn was forty-five and had been married for six years to a man she found selfish, miserly, and childish. She held herself back until she could no longer contain herself, and then complained bitterly to him. He responded by avoiding her, and she ended up feeling worse. Evelyn regarded her situation as hopeless and was considering divorce, but she worried about supporting herself and being alone. Diagnostically, she was hard to classify. She was unhappy but not a depressive; she functioned well at home and at work; and her main symptom was her marriage. She wanted to try Prozac to see if it would alleviate her unhappiness and calm her rage at her husband. This was the kind of situation that I found difficult. There was no clear psychiatric illness; Evelyn did not even have a subsyndromal illness. As a clinician, I felt vulnerable to the charge that I was a pill-pusher, a psychiatric protector of the status quo (Evelyn's marriage), the kind of doctor who drugged women so they would overlook or not respond to mistreatment at the hands of men—in this case, Evelyn's husband.

Two considerations made me go ahead with Prozac. The first rule of medicine is "do no harm." The harm to this woman, whom I had seen for months in psychotherapy and had been unable to help, was to leave her in unnecessary pain. Second, doctors often have to act without a complete diagnosis. When all diagnostic explorations fail, the surgeon may be forced to open the abdomen for exploratory purposes. The orthopedist, unable to discover the source of back pain, may prescribe medication, a change in diet, and exercise. The allergist, unable to find the reason for red and itchy eyes, may offer drops. I had a patient in pain and no diagnosis, and decided to proceed. This may seem irresponsible to the ethicist, but necessary to the clinician with a patient in pain.

Prozac produced a curious result in Evelyn. She was able to hold back her sharp, impulsive retorts at her childish, selfish husband, and to consider what effect her words might have on him, and how best to get him to do what she wanted. She decided she would get much further with her egotist if she flattered him and seemed grateful for all he had done for her. It worked like a charm. He began to come home earlier, and even offered to help by doing the dishes. Her marriage became much happier. Furthermore, she was able to observe this sequence of events and learn from it. The idea that one either gains insight in psychotherapy or is cured by Prozac is a false dichotomy set up by those involved in a debate. When emotions are in control, people can learn for themselves through experience or with the help of a therapist.

The Antidepressants and Suicide

Once again, the alleged association between the antidepressants and suicide has been raised, this time resulting in the FDA considering a recommendation that manufacturers print a warning label stating that medicated depressed patients, especially children, be carefully monitored. It is my belief that all psychiatric patients, medicated or not, be given the full attention of those responsible for their treatment.

Nothing is more terrible than the suicide of any person, but it is especially terrible in the case of a child. Parents are devastated, as are siblings, friends, classmates, and teachers. Psychiatrists, therapists, family physicians—no one is spared the trauma.

Naturally, questions arise in the aftermath of a suicide. Could it have been predicted? Who or what is to blame? How can we prevent it in the future? Then the answers come. It is the doctor's fault for not being vigilant. It is the school that failed to pay attention. The parents are too busy and too preoccupied. Finally, some charge the medication itself. How could something designed to prevent such tragedy be the cause? It is natural and human to want to find a cause, place the blame, and prevent tragedy from happening again.

Do antidepressants cause suicide, however infrequent the occurrence? Should no child or adolescent take them, even though one million currently do? Is there proof that they are effective so that the benefit outweighs the risk? I'm afraid the definitive research hasn't been done to prove either their efficacy or their danger. It's been said that doctors make life and death decisions based on inadequate evidence. I am afraid this assertion is true. The FDA is right to urge prescribers to pay close attention.

Twenty years ago when the government and the Veteran's Administration were supporting multiple studies, unlike now when only minimal clinical research is done by drug companies before they bring new products to market, I reviewed with several of my psychiatric residents the then available literature to see if antidepressants prevented suicide. We found that they do not. Our study was never accepted for publication, allegedly because of design flaws, but I also suspect psychiatric journals did not want to have it enshrined in print that these medications did not prevent suicide. Unfortunately, we did not look at whether they caused suicide, but others have and never discovered any statistical relationship between SSRIs and suicide.

More than 20 million people have taken antidepressants in the United States alone, and some of them have killed themselves. Every death is tragic, but no proof exists to demonstrate that the drugs were to blame. People commit suicide for many reasons. No one single cause prompts them to take this step.

Would I allow a member of my family to take an antidepressant? Yes. Would I watch them closely, especially if I suspected a danger of suicide? Absolutely! Do I think antidepressants *cause* suicide? I do not. Most psychiatrists agree with my position. A few do not.

Can Prozac Make People Worse?

Prozac can make someone worse if that person becomes manic, paranoid, has a seizure, develops a skin rash, or has a bad interaction with another drug. These dangers have been covered in the preceding section on SSRIs.

It is in the area of personality and temperament that the most interesting changes for the worse occur. It is a rule of medicine that every treatment which has an effect also produces a side effect. Thus, if the meek can be empowered, they can be made too much so, while the assertive can become lacking in sensitivity and tact, excessively forward and brash. If the irritable and rageful can be calmed, then they can be made too meek, while the normally assertive may become too forgiving.

Finally, there is the problem of the incomplete cure. If the psychiatrist monitors the patient for side effects, it is also necessary to carefully watch for the partial failure to recover, for in this category lies much misery and loss of capacity to function. Partially recovered depressives suffer largely unrecognized and unhelped by their physicians.

The following are three cases illustrating Prozac failures, in the meek, the rageful, and the depressed:

Frank

Forty-nine-year-old Frank had been a machinist until several years ago when he decided to try to become an engineer. He took courses and tests qualifying him to assume this role. During his long, bitter divorce, he suffered a major depressive episode. He was put on Prozac, and it sped his recovery. He decided to remain on it while he interviewed for a new job.

It was during his description of an interview that I realized that this normally sensitive and cautious man was being harmed by Prozac. He felt the interviewer was trying to trick him in order to test him. Normally Frank would have noticed this and handled himself and the interviewer skillfully. Instead he said, "I'm not going to fall for that one," and openly discussed the trap he felt was being set. The interviewer said nothing, but I was not surprised when Frank was turned down.

Frank could be labeled either hypomanic due to Prozac, or a previously undiagnosed bipolar, whose brashness was due to pressure of speech and grandiosity, and his desire to become an engineer inspired by an elevated mood. But his mood was not "clearly different" from his normal one, and if his ambition to improve himself were grandiosity, then everyone seeking a job promotion must be sick. His thoughts were not racing; he was not distractible, agitated, sleepless, involved in buying sprees, sexual indiscretions, or foolish investments. I did not think him hypomanic. What I did think was that Frank had been tipped by Prozac from being sensitive to being insensitive, from considering the consequences of his behavior to being oblivious, and from being normally cautious to being impulsive.

Barbara

Forty-one-year-old Barbara divorced after ten years of marriage. She became accustomed to living alone and enjoyed her job. But she was given to outbursts of temper, and this, plus her chronic boredom and dissatisfaction, led to her being placed on Prozac. As a consequence, her relationships with her brothers, sisters, and parents vastly improved. She tolerated their faults much better, and stopped hanging up phones and walking angrily out of rooms. She was very grateful for Prozac's calming effect on her previously tempestuous family ties. Unfortunately, the Prozac effect went too far.

Barbara met an unemployed woman, became friendly, and let her move in. She supported her, let her use the car, and did whatever she asked. Her new roommate would criticize and ridicule Barbara virtually nonstop, stay out overnight without notice or explanation, and refuse to keep her company on weekends. Finally, after a year of verbal abuse and inconsiderate behavior, Barbara asked her to leave. Several months later, when off Prozac, she described how the drug not only had calmed her rages but had made her too tranquil, willing to tolerate her former roommate's freeloading and harassment, something she would never have permitted when off the drug.

Joyce

Joyce was forty-seven years old, married, with three children. She had been chronically depressed for over twenty years, the last six of which she had been on 20 to 60 mg of Prozac, depending upon the severity of her chronically moderate depression. When it was at its worst, psychotic thoughts entered her mind, and she began to feel the neighbors were talking about her and saying uncomplimentary things.

If we measured Joyce's condition using the Hamilton Depression Scale (see pages 43–44), Joyce would be considered improved, perhaps even cured, after taking Prozac. But only one of the seventeen items on the scale involves work and interests, which means one could be scored as nondepressed, yet not work or have any interests. I believe that almost all drug studies contain this weakness in the Hamilton scale, one that is slowly being recognized by researchers interested in social adjustment and quality of life following depression.

Social Adjustment After Prozac

Prozac moves most people in the right direction, but it is very important to think about where you are starting from. If you are severely depressed, it will take longer for you to respond than if you are mildly ill. Prozac successes among the timid, irritable, fatigued, abusive, and insecure who do not have major depression are gratifying for doctor and patient. Giovanni Cassano et al. studied social adjustment in 176 patients with mild to moderate depression. They found that those on tricyclic antidepressants who reported improvement were able to work and felt well, but their relationships with spouses and children remained impaired, and they participated in few leisure and social activities. These researchers suggested that impairment in the capacity to enjoy leisure may remain constant during some depressed people's lifetimes. I have seen this happen with certain chronically depressed people on Prozac, too. Some recover their leisure and social interests very slowly, long after the rest of their depressed symptoms have disappeared. Others, unfortunately, are able to work and carry out the tasks necessary in their lives but have no hobbies, interests, or passions. These are the loners, the workaholics, and the idle shut-ins. This is the main reason why most depressives need more than drugs to be truly cured. They need help getting along with their spouses, children, neighbors, and friends, and in finding activities that will give them pleasure.

Dr. William Coryell et al. studied 148 bipolar and 240 unipolar affective disorder patients at the time they sought treatment and again five years later, and compared their overall functioning to that of their nondepressed relatives. In their report, Dr. Coryell and his colleagues noted the "enduring psychosocial consequences of mania and depression" and found that five years after the onset of illness, the depressed were less likely to be employed and to have been promoted at work, and more likely to have lower incomes. In addition, unipolar and bipolar patients were only half as likely to have ever been married, and those married were twice as often divorced or separated. The unipolars who remained married were unhappy both with their marriage and with their sex lives. Dr. Coryell's group found the impairment of seemingly recovered depressives to remain serious: their job status and incomes continued to decline; their marriages were still miserable, and their sexual relationships unhappy. The authors note that their sample of depressed subjects may have been sicker on average, and thus more chronically impaired, for they were recruited from five specialized care centers. They question the usual practice of defining recovery from depression in terms of an absence of symptoms, while overlooking profound psychosocial damage.

While the detriment may grow less the longer the person is symptom-free, these authors believe impairment to be life-long in many cases.

We need more studies of the effects of major depression on marriage, work, and leisure-time activities. While many people recover fully, many others require much more than the symptomatic relief provided by Prozac. They need help with their jobs, marriages, sexual functioning, friendships, and with their leisure-time activities. Work and pleasure must also improve, not just the other sixteen items on the Hamilton Depression Scale.

Prozac's Interactions with Other Drugs

Although I have discussed this subject generally in the section on SSRIs, I wish to bring it up again here with respect to Prozac for two reasons. It is the subject of intense interest and recent research, and because Prozac lingers in the body for weeks, it affects not only those drugs you already are on but those you may take in the future. Thus, five weeks must elapse after you stop taking Prozac before you can start the MAOIs, Nardil, or Parnate. While MAOIs, L-tryptophan, and the anti–Parkinson's disease drug L-deprenyl (Eldepryl) must *never* be taken along with Prozac, other drugs can and will be, but it is necessary to know how they will be affected. For example, the effect of the tricyclic antidepressant desipramine will be increased many times by Prozac. Thus, when combined with Prozac, desipramine must be used in a lower than normal dosage. To a lesser extent, Prozac magnifies the effect of Valium and Xanax. Prozac also increases the effect of Clozaril, and therefore the risk of seizure associated with the latter.

The effect of Prozac on these other drugs is mediated through Prozac's effect on liver metabolism. No one knows whether long-term use of Prozac will harm the liver. Up to now, however, Prozac does not seem especially toxic to the liver.

Taking Prozac for the Rest of Your Life

There are two types of major depressives: those people who suffer only from depression, and those who suffer from mania and depression. The first typically have four to six episodes in their lifetime; the bipolars, seven to nine periods of acute illness. Furthermore, unipolar episodes occur closer together and become more severe and long-lasting as the person gets older. One study at the University of Pittsburgh found that half of unipolar and bipolar depressives who stop taking their medication relapse in one year. Furthermore, the older a person is when suffering a first episode, the more likely there will be a recurrence in two years. Therefore, I would advise severe major depressives who have had three episodes, those over age forty who have had two episodes, and those over age fifty who have had one episode, to remain on an SSRI for life. Another reason for long-term Prozac use is the presence of residual symptoms following an acute episode or the presence of incapacitating dysthymia. I realize that taking Prozac continuously carries unknown risks, which I hope will not be serious, but severe major depressive disorder is also serious, recurs, and requires continuous medication for its prevention.

As for those taking Prozac for milder but nonetheless painful and limiting emotional states, I would suggest trying to come off the medication after a year or two. Although whatever it was that made you start taking Prozac may come back, the symptom-free period in between may have helped you acquire new social and stress-reducing skills, either with or without a psychotherapist, and you may find that you no longer need Prozac. If this is not the case, go back on it, but with the intention of doing so for a limited time only. I have seen many people outgrow their need for Prozac. Only the severe major depressive needs it for life.

When discontinuing use of Prozac, do so gradually. If you are on more than one capsule, reduce it by one every few weeks. Once you are down to one capsule a day, start to space it out to every other, and then every third, day. The reason for this is that if you stop taking the drug suddenly, you may become anxious or depressed, or feel unwell and mistake this for proof that you still need Prozac. In fact, what you are experiencing is a withdrawal reaction. I used to think that because Prozac lasts for weeks in the system, gradual withdrawal should be unnecessary, but I have seen people develop unpleasant symptoms from the sudden withdrawal of the drug.

Severe PMS (Premenstrual Syndrome) and the More Symptomatic Premenstrual Dysphoric Disorder (PMDD)

The *American Psychiatric Press Textbook of Psychiatry* (2d ed., 1994) notes that "both men and women attribute negative psychological states and behaviors in women to the menstrual cycle" and laments the lack of good diagnostic criteria and treatment for this condition. Thus, there is great controversy surrounding the use of Prozac for treating premenstrual syndrome.

Dr. Barbara Parry, a professor of psychiatry at the University of California at San Diego, writes that in PMS "the mood and behavioral changes are recurrent and predictable." These changes can be divided into mood and bodily complaints. The mood changes include depression, fatigue, anxiety, tension, irritability, and headache. The bodily changes include abdominal bloating, breast tenderness, and ankle swelling. Dr. Parry reviews a long list of mostly unsatisfactory attempts to treat PMS. Open trials of various drugs initially look promising, only to prove ineffective when subjected to controlled, double-blind review.

One double-blind study of PMS by Dr. Andrea Stone (1991) found Prozac to be effective in treating both the mood and physical symptoms associated with PMS. But even in this carefully designed study, which by its rigor was able to eliminate placebo responders, 50 percent had a history of major depression. Nonetheless, women whose PMS was sufficiently severe as to seriously interfere with their social or occupational functioning were helped. A larger, but less rigorous, double-blind study reported by Dr. Meir Steiner in the *New England Journal of Medicine* (June 8, 1995) also found Prozac to be more effective than a placebo.

A large multicenter controlled trial of Zoloft by Kimberly Yonkers in 1997 showed the drug to be effective in relieving depressive symptoms, physical discomfort, and irritability in PMDD. Several other studies also found Zoloft effective. An SSRI taken only during the two weeks before severe PMS occurs is possibly as useful as taking the drug throughout the month. Sarafem (2000), a pink and purple pill pushed to treat PMDD, is not a new drug; it is Prozac.

Who Should Start on Less Than 20 mg of Prozac a Day?

In 1988, when Prozac was released in the United States, only 20-mg capsules were available, forcing many on the drug to open the capsules, pour the contents into cranberry juice, leave the mixture in the refrigerator, and drink half one day and half the next. After complaints and several years of "cranzac," the 10-mg capsule and the liquid form were released. In 1999 a 10-mg scored tablet was made available. The existence of only a 20-mg capsule initially had an important positive effect, in that it forced people to be on a full therapeutic dose from the start. In spite of subsequent refinements, there seems to be something almost magical about the 20-mg dose, and debate continues among experts who think a dose of 40 to 80 mg makes more people better than does 20 mg, and those who find no advantage—the so-called flat dose response curve. Since many who received the older tricyclics were on too low a dosage, Prozac helped many more people because it was given in adequate amounts.

There are three kinds of people who should start on less than 20 mg a day. First, those who suffer panic attacks or who are very anxious in general, who may find the SSRI side effects of nervousness, insomnia, and anxiety intolerable. A lower dosage (5 mg) allows you to become accustomed to the drug gradually, and then the dosage can be raised. The other two kinds of people who should be started on less than 20 mg are the elderly, who metabolize and excrete the drug more slowly, and those with liver or kidney disease. Prozac is effective in the elderly, although no more so than any other SSRI, and causes fewer side effects than the tricyclics. It increases the blood levels of other antidepressants, which should therefore be used in lower than normal dosages.

If you elect to begin Prozac at 10 mg or less, and are in good medical health, and if you are not bothered by side effects, then it is wise to increase the dose to 20 mg after a week. Although some people may not need this, most do, and it will speed the response. Depression is painful, and the sooner gone, the better. There is a small percentage (under 10 percent) who metabolize Prozac slowly, and they may require lower dosage.

Double Depression and Prozac

Chronic depression of varying severity punctuated by episodes of acute major depression is called double depression. This concept is important because it used to be thought that acute major depression was self-limited and followed by complete recovery, and now it is known that about 20 percent do not recover completely. These people are candidates for continuous Prozac treatment, which not only shortens and diminishes the intensity of the acute episode but also can relieve the impairment associated with chronic double depression.

Childhood and Adolescent Depression and Prozac

Since 1950, there has been an increased rate of depression in children and adolescents. Major depression in young people is a chronic and recurring condition, so that 40 percent suffer a second depressive episode within two years, and 70 percent in five years. These children and adolescents are

118 THE NEW ANTIDEPRESSANTS AND ANTIANXIETIES

affected in their school performance and in their relationships with peers and family. They are also likely to have conduct disorders and conflicts with their mothers and fathers. The condition persists into adulthood and continues to affect their work, social, and family life. There is a high risk of suicide in the young depressed group.

Despite several attempts at placebo-controlled studies of antidepressants in child and adolescent depression, no difference has been found between the effects of the drug and those of the placebo. Unfortunately, no psychotherapy or drug therapy of early-onset depression has been effective in unipolar or bipolar children or adolescents. Nonetheless, Prozac and other antidepressants are widely used in depressed young people by clinicians who believe them to be effective. There is no general consensus as to which children are most likely to benefit at what dose and how long they should be treated. Children and adolescents do respond well to Prozac; it is just that they respond well to a placebo, too, and it is this high placebo response rate that makes it so difficult to establish Prozac's superiority over a sugar pill. Since childhood and adolescent depression often progresses into adult depression, it may just be that when young these individuals are more influenced by the promise of any pill. However, in severe childhood and adolescent depression, neither Prozac nor a placebo seems to do much good.

The question of administering antidepressant drugs to adolescents, or even worse to young children, and whether the drugs increase the number of suicides, has recently made headlines. The data upon which these serious charges rest is allegedly hidden in drug company files, which the United States Congress plans to compel be opened, provided they exist and have not been destroyed.

A National Institute of Mental Health–supported study by Barbara Geller, M.D., et al., from the Department of Psychiatry, Washington University in St. Louis, appearing in the prestigious *Archives of General Psychiatry* in May of 2004, reveals the primitive state of psychiatric knowledge on the subject of severely ill children with mood disorders. The conclusion was that "long-episode" chronic childhood mania exists. Eighty-six children whose disorder began, on average, at age seven and one-half remained ill for one to two years. To look at the list of what was wrong with this group of prepubertal and early onset adolescent children with mania is overwhelming. Not only were most of them manic, they also exhibited:

Poor judgment (90%)—e.g., hypersexuality, daredevil acts, silliness, uninhibited people-seeking
Irritable mood (98%)
Distractibility (93%)
Major depression (55%)
Dysthymia (34%)
Psychosis (60%)
Suicidality (25%)
Attention deficit/hyperactivity disorder (ADHD) (86%)
Oppositional defiant (78%)

Looking at this list makes me wonder whether the condition could be better named "severely ill psychiatric disordered children" rather than mania, since most of them are also depressed, psychotic, and suffering from ADHD and conduct disorder (oppositional defiant), and 25 percent are suicidal (how severely and lethally the study did not specify).

Since this was a "natural history of mania" study and made no mention of treatment, most of which I assume was tried and failed, to pick out Prozac and define it or any other SSRI as the culprit seems to me on the face of it as impossible. It is well known that there is a correlation between the severity of psychiatric disorder and successful suicide. In fact, while 15 percent of severe depressives kill themselves, so do 13 percent of schizophrenics.

The labels the FDA is considering that psychiatric patients on antidepressants should be carefully followed by their doctors needs the emphasis it is now receiving. All psychiatric patients, in fact all medical patients, need the watchful, caring eye of a physician who knows them well. "Take two of these pills and e-mail me in the morning" may be the subject of a *New Yorker* cartoon, but it is not proper medicine.

At this time, the study of depression at both ends of the age spectrum, the young and the old, is intense. We need more answers in both areas. I hope they will come soon. Until then, Prozac is worth a try, but produces no miracles.

Prozac in Acute Bipolar Depression

The danger of antidepressant drug use in bipolar patients is mood destabilization with hypomania or rapid cycling (four or more episodes of mania or depression in a twelve-month period) or both. Thus, once the depression is relieved, the antidepressant is withdrawn, and the mood-stabilizing drug is continued alone. Because Prozac has a very long stay in the body, so that the blood level declines by only a half in two weeks, it may make sense to use a shorter-acting SSRI in bipolar people in case hypomania occurs. Whether antidepressants actually induce mania in bipolar patients or the manic phase is a product of the disease itself (and not drug-caused) has never been adequately researched, and most likely will never be because it would be necessary to deny treatment to half of the depressed bipolar patients, who would be on a placebo.

Prozac in Atypical Depression

The atypical depressive eats and sleeps too much, and is irritable, agitated, oversensitive to rejection, unresponsive to gladdening events, and experiences heaviness in the limbs. The oversensitivity to rejection arises in youth and remains throughout most of adult life. It is present both when the person is and is not depressed. Those who are oversensitive to rejection cannot stand criticism at work or from friends and family. Younger people are more likely to exhibit atypical features. Oversensitivity to rejection can interfere with long-term relationships, making them stormy or totally disrupting them, and those so afflicted may avoid intimacy out of fear of being hurt. It also interferes with their relationships with supervisors and others at work.

Studies have repeatedly shown that atypical depressives respond better to the MAOIs Nardil and Parnate than they do to the tricyclic antidepressants Elavil and Tofranil. The SSRIs are currently thought to be as effective, and are likely to be used first, and the MAOIs reserved only for when the SSRIs fail.

Claire is an example of someone with atypical depression. She is forty-three and is getting divorced after ten years of a stormy marriage. She spent most of those years in therapy complaining about her husband's insensitivity and how it hurt her. She has many women friends and goes to one with tales of mistreatment at the hands of the other. Claire spends hours thinking about what an acquaintance said or did, about a party she went to or to which she was not invited. She prides herself on being sensitive. In fact, she suffers a lot and is oversensitive. At a time when she was depressed and furious with her best friend, she agreed to try Prozac. After several weeks, she began to feel better; her mind was no longer preoccupied with the snubs and wounds she suffered. She became more productive at work and more content with the people in her life.

Prozac and Melancholia

Melancholia is a severe form of depression in which the person experiences complete loss of pleasure and is not cheered up even when something good happens. The melancholic's mood is distinctly different from normal sadness, such as that resulting from the death of a loved one. The depressed mood is worse in the morning; the sufferer wakes up at 2 to 4 A.M. unable to return to sleep, is agitated or slowed, loses a lot of weight, has no appetite, and feels excessive guilt. Melancholics may need hospitalization, and their recovery with antidepressant medication is slow, requiring weeks or months. There is debate over whether the older tricyclic antidepressants are more effective than the SSRIs in treating melancholia, and more studies will be needed to settle it.

Prozac and Euphoria

Euphoria is a feeling of great happiness or well-being, and derives from the Greek word *euphoros*, relating to good health. Prozac is not listed as a cause of euphoria in the American Psychiatric Association's textbook (1994), while alcohol-, cocaine-, and methadone-induced euphoria are. In the *PDR*, euphoria is described as occurring infrequently (1 in 100 to 1 in 1,000) among those on Prozac. Dr. Lars F. Gram, in a review of Prozac in the *New England Journal of Medicine* (November 17, 1994), ends by saying, "The published data on the antidepressant effect of fluoxetine [Prozac] do not fully explain its popularity. One may speculate that fluoxetine has psychobiologic effects not strictly related to the biology of depression and that it acts primarily as a mood-or-affect-modulating agent." Does this mean euphoria, and if so, is this good or bad? If one has enthusiasm for a subject or a cause, feels great excitement and interest, is one manic or to be envied? If you have lost all interest in things and are suffering from a melancholic depression, should euphoria be viewed as a return of health or a sickness? Do you really feel great interest and excitement in what you are doing or are you merely high from a pill? Are you in love or the victim of a love potion? The line between feeling well and being slightly manic can be unclear.

The *DSM* IV describes the elevated mood characteristic of a manic episode as "euphoric, unusually good, cheerful, or high . . . [and] it is recognized as excessive by those who know the person well." It then goes on to describe the enthusiasm as "indiscriminate" and the accompanying self-esteem as "inflated," even grandiose. The mood, according to the *DSM* IV must be abnormally elevated for at least a week. I will not repeat here the earlier sections on manic and hypomanic episodes, but will only say that Prozac, in my experience, induces what I would call a "healthy" euphoria or feeling of confidence, well-being, and enthusiasm in a significant percentage of the people I treat with it, and in a small minority an excessive high, one in which their loved ones find them abnormally excited by routine events. This latter hypomanic group presents a diagnostic problem if they live alone and are not sufficiently intimate with anyone for their excitement about the routine to be called to their (or a physician's) attention, because they run the risk of unintentionally alienating coworkers and customers with their brash and insensitive behavior. When an individual becomes clinically manic, it is easy for strangers to spot; the hypomanic's expansive or irritable mood, distractibility, excessive activity, and talkativeness may be more difficult for others to distinguish as abnormal. It is this latter continuum from healthy euphoria to mild hypomania that the individual who crosses that line will not notice for himself, and he will end up suffering the social and occupational consequences. Hypomanics can be energetic, cheerful, productive, and enjoyable to be around, but they can also be disorganized, distractible, irritable, and lacking in social judgment—attributes into which they have no insight and which can get them in trouble at home and on the job. When I noted earlier that Prozac is not a euphoriant, I should have added a qualifier. I should have said that Prozac is often a healthy euphoriant and only occasionally causes loss of judgment and abnormal euphoria (hypomania).

"Me, Too" Drugs

Eli Lilly and Co.'s 1998 Prozac sales were $2.8 billion, leading other drug companies to market new entries in the SSRI class. A "me, too" drug is a similar product that competes for the same group of patients. The companies then promote the drugs aggressively in an attempt to distinguish their own, even though they can, in fact, barely be told apart. These efforts are aimed at physicians, pharmacists, and sometimes directly at the public. Because Prozac has been such a phenomenal success since 1988, Zoloft (1992), Paxil (1993), Luvox (1995), Celexa (1999), and Lexapro (2003) have followed. If any of these were to take away even 10 percent of the Prozac share, it would mean $250 million in sales. There are some advantages to the availability of "me, too" drugs. If a person is allergic to one, the presence of a second SSRI in the form of a different chemical compound to which he is not allergic is an advantage. If the side effects are slightly different, one SSRI may be tolerated, while another is not. Since 15 to 20 percent of people discontinue use of their first SSRI because of side effects and another 20 percent stop because they are not being helped, it is useful to have an alternative available.

In spite of a mythology regarding how SSRIs differ, here is a list of their basic similarities:

- All of the SSRIs are equally effective.
- All can be taken once a day (except Luvox in doses over 100 mg).
- One pill daily is usually enough. (Thus, an effective dose can be used from the beginning of treatment.)
- All require days to weeks before they begin to work.
- All prevent relapse equally well.
- An overdose of any of the SSRIs is much safer on the heart.
- Their side effects are much more alike than different. What few differences there are will be discussed under each drug.

Since no SSRI is more effective or better tolerated than Prozac, manufacturers have emphasized differences in duration of action, metabolism, age effect, ease in altering blood level, and reduced risk of drug interactions as selling points. Because Prozac and its active metabolite are only half gone in two weeks, whereas Zoloft and Paxil half disappear in one day, all kinds of sinister things can be imagined about Prozac. It can drive mania and interact with MAOIs. So, of course, can the other SSRIs, but maybe less so. Unfortunately, the advantage of Zoloft and Paxil in mania is unproven and the need to wait two weeks, versus five weeks for Prozac, before beginning an MAOI rarely comes up. Prozac dosage is harder to adjust than the other two, but this is a theoretical and rarely a clinical problem. When doubt arises about what is a drug side effect (e.g., headache, lethargy), the answer lies in the clinical decision either to maintain the dose to see if the side effect goes away, or to cut the amount. The solution to the problem is no more instantly clear with Zoloft than with Prozac.

The disadvantages of a longer-acting drug are emphasized by those advocating Zoloft, but actually it is the fears of it that rule. The advantages of Prozac are that people may forget to take their drug one day, or fail to fill their prescription. Prozac remains in the body, while Zoloft does not. A once-weekly 90-mg fluoxetine was made available in 2001 for maintenance treatment only for people stabilized on 20 mg per day. It can also be used in patients stabilized on other SSRIs, such as Celexa, Paxil, or Zoloft.

The Attacks on Prozac

Now that Prozac resides in the old-age home of generics, we have a chance to review the furor that has surrounded it. The legal department of Eli Lilly has fielded over one hundred cases. Although the company was well paid for its trouble, I think it would help the reader to pause and review the near-hysterical cultural wars waged over whether this drug was a savior or a poison. At times the tone reached biblical proportion, joined into by scientologists, the government, medical experts, conspiracy theorists, capitalists and socialists, the therapy industry, HMOs, the insurance industry, and patients' rights groups. Prozac provided a Rorschach test on which was projected attitudes about illness, character, biology, and free will.

There are two groups of charges mounted against this beacon designed to safely lead people out of depression to the light of health and productivity. I will begin with the less serious accusations. There are those surrounding its birth in sin, the ones reporting that Eli Lilly distorted the research, substituting euphemisms for serious side effects such as suicidal impulses, and suppressing studies, only publishing those favorable to the drug's effectiveness. I do not wish to imply that such charges are entirely false and trivial, but merely to question the shrill tone in which they were delivered. The accusation that Prozac made a significant number of depressed people suicidal or homicidal came early, was oft repeated, and occupied the deliberations of courtrooms, the FDA, and serious researchers. The verdict was repeatedly reached: not guilty, but even now the doubt lingers in the minds of some.

Prozac occasionally loses its effectiveness, sometimes within months, colloquially called the "poop out" phenomenon, and variously attributed to either tolerance (becoming less responsive to a previously effective dose) or to the loss of what was, in fact, a placebo improvement. This can be fixed often by merely raising the dose. The term tolerance is also used to account for the abuse of illicit drugs and the need to escalate a narcotic in order to elicit the same high. Other subliminal narcotic references applied to Prozac include a withdrawal syndrome following the sudden cessation of the drug, or especially the other shorter-acting SSRIs, which causes nausea, vertigo, flulike symptoms, mood swings, and irritability. This guilt by association has been especially successful against the benzodiazepines, which will be reviewed elsewhere in this book. But in the case of Prozac, people almost never seek higher doses, and certainly not to stave off withdrawal symptoms, behaviors common to opiate addicts. It is safe to say that the sudden termination of any psychoactive drug that has been taken over months or years is a dangerous practice leading to painful consequences.

Sexual dysfunction was deliberately downplayed by Eli Lilly, antagonists charge. The four-to-six-week prerelease study does not inquire actively about sexual side effects, and thus severely depressed patients, especially women, say nothing about them. The less than 5 percent commonly reported explodes to 60 percent or more in follow-up studies, giving proof to the original deceit. There are many other plausible explanations for this besides illegal cover-up. Deeply depressed patients are in a lot of pain, and not thinking about their sex lives, something that resumes its importance when they recover. Estimates of sexual disturbances run about 30 percent in the general population, still higher in untreated depressives, and thus, the addition by Prozac is not as great as it seems on the surface. Nonetheless, it is real, and it presents a problem, causing many people who would otherwise benefit to stop taking it.

A syndrome affecting motivation and causing severe fatigue has also been attributed to Prozac. Since lack of energy and desire to move are also characteristic of deep depression, this distinction is a hard one.

Serious Charges Against Prozac

I do not wish to imply that the preceding was not serious. Perhaps this section should be labeled "Prozac as Poison." In general, this assault on the drug stems from an exaggeration of what the critics say already exists, and an even more frightening augur of yet unknown serious problems to come. References to the delay in discovering the serious, initially hidden, damaging effects of Thorazine on the central nervous system are invoked. And Prozac is convicted, it seems to me, by the McCarthy-like tactic of guilt by association. The problem with this attack is that Thorazine affects dopamine, and Prozac serotonin; that Thorazine used in high doses for long periods results in a significant incidence of the facial tics and sometimes more violent general thrashing movements of tardive dyskinesia; and Prozac almost never causes them, no matter what its dose and duration. Other false analogies to cocaine, ecstasy (MDMA), and Redux (a diet pill withdrawn in 1997) are also occasionally invoked in the charges against Prozac. Having reviewed the literature, the testimony before the FDA, and the pronouncements of experts, I believe Prozac to be a safe drug. Of course, it has had plenty of defense by Lilly's army of lawyers, along with its powerful marketing, sales force, and advertising arms. The generic benzodiazepines have no such strong defenders, and lie convicted without a fight. I will try in a later section to come to their aid, not to serve as a judge and exonerate them, but in an attempt to restore some rhetorical balance to the debate so far dominated by the directors of addiction psychiatry, addiction medicine, chemical dependency, and collectively referred to sometimes as "addictionologists."

Drugs of Abuse

The physicians deemed addiction experts are supported by that terrifying governmental agency, the Drug Enforcement Administration of the United States Department of Justice, which issues a Controlled Substance Registration Certificate every two years to all physicians whom they deem in good standing. The states also register Controlled Substances Practitioners. These agencies divide all drugs according to their potential for abuse. Schedule I has no recognized medical use (e.g., heroin). Schedule II permits a thirty-day supply, is nonrefillable, and includes morphine, oxycodone, Ritalin, and Dexedrine. Schedule III permits a thirty-day supply, is refillable five times in six months, and includes the barbiturates. Schedule IV has no limit on monthly tablet number, is refillable five times in six months, and includes the benzodiazepines. Schedules V and VI have no limits for amount or number of refills, and encompass other drugs, including the antidepressants. Thus, the SSRIs are legally recognized as less addicting than the benzodiazepines. Whether or not this is true is something I will discuss later.

Prozac is neither the miracle ending depression and other forms of human suffering that it seemed to be in 1987 at its launch, nor the poison charged by its detractors. It is a good, solid addition to the physician's power to help millions of suffering people around the world. We are fortunate to have it.

Zoloft

The annual sales of Pfizer's Zoloft (approved in 1992) are now $2.5 billion. The modern antidepressants are the most commonly purchased prescription drugs. One half of a dose of Zoloft is excreted by the body in one day (Prozac takes one to two weeks). The two top-selling antidepressants now are Zoloft (sertraline) and Paxil (paroxetine), Prozac having slipped badly since its cheaper generic versions became available. The armies of drug salespeople no longer pitch Prozac, leaving the field open to the other two. Paxil, however, has just been made available in generic form, and Zoloft will soon follow.

How Does Zoloft Work?

Zoloft reaches maximum concentration in the blood five to eight hours after being ingested, a process aided if the patient takes it with food. Whenever a person starts a new intermediate- to long-acting drug, the blood level rises over days to weeks until such time as a so-called steady state occurs, in which the concentration of the drug in the body remains on a plateau, an equilibrium between the daily dose ingested and bodily excretion of the medication. Because it is metabolized faster than Prozac, a steady concentration of Zoloft is reached in the body in one week rather than two to eight weeks. Steady-state blood levels are reached within five half-lives. Sertraline's twenty-four-hour half-life predicts a steady-state blood level after five days. If a second pill must be added because of a failure to respond, the blood level of Zoloft adjusts within one week. This point regarding the speed of blood level adjustment is made much of by Zoloft advocates, although I fail to see the value of it. No one has claimed that Zoloft cures the patient faster or even that the blood levels of SSRIs have any connection to the number of patients who respond. Perhaps there is some advantage to Zoloft's being 97 percent cleared from the body one week after the patient stops taking the drug, whereas Prozac is only half gone in over two weeks, but even here, this is counterbalanced by the disadvantage of having to taper off the Zoloft dose more carefully to avoid withdrawal reactions.

Most SSRI research has been done on outpatients, and thus there has been concern about whether these drugs are as effective as the tricyclics in severe, inpatient depressives. In a large controlled Danish study, severely depressed inpatients responded better to a tricyclic (clomipramine) in comparison to the SSRIs Paxil and Celexa. The new serotonin and norepinephrine reuptake inhibitor Effexor (released in 1994) was found to be superior to Prozac in two studies of severely depressed patients. More research on the SSRIs' effectiveness in depressed inpatients is necessary, but their equal efficacy to tricyclics in outpatients has been established.

SSRIs cause the side effects of agitation, anxiety, and insomnia. Thus, there is concern about how people with a mixture of anxiety and depression or those with recurrent insomnia will be affected. Zoloft has been effective in both the anxious and the sleepless. Neither the severity nor the chronicity of depression diminished the effectiveness of Zoloft, which can be given over a lifetime where necessary.

Dosage

Most people begin taking Zoloft at 50 mg once daily, either in the morning or in the evening. The therapeutic effect is apparent within two to four weeks, as it is with other antidepressants. After a month, if there is little response, the dose is raised by 50 mg per week until a maximum of 200 mg daily is reached. People with liver or kidney disease or those who are elderly take lower amounts.

Side Effects

As with Prozac, Zoloft can cause headaches, nausea (33 percent), diarrhea (25 percent), insomnia, but less agitation and anxiety. A mild tremor occurs in up to 20 percent of people taking Zoloft, as it does in those taking Prozac and lithium. Dizziness is also fairly common. Like Prozac, Zoloft has little effect on the heart, and thus is much safer than tricyclics in overdosage. Since the threat of suicide always exists in depression, the safety of the SSRIs with respect to possible overdose is particularly important. Zoloft causes less dry mouth, drowsiness, fatigue, dizziness, constipation, and weight gain than the tricyclics.

Efforts to distinguish Zoloft from Prozac on the basis of side effects have not been very successful, as the two drugs are more alike than different. However, Prozac is more activating than Zoloft. In fact, Zoloft does not exceed placebo in anxiety or agitation side effects. All the SSRIs produce similar sexual dysfunction. Side effects of all the SSRIs are dose related, so that it makes sense to take the least amount required for a good clinical response. Since it takes two to four weeks for there to be any improvement, and many more before complete recovery, it is advisable to be patient and not to keep upping the dose during this time, especially since studies of elevation reveal that the same percentage of patients recover on 50 mg as on 200 mg, but many more on 200 mg are uncomfortable from side effects.

As mentioned earlier in describing the report of Drs. Brown and Harrison (see page 72), 79 percent of those who discontinued use of Prozac because of side effects were able to complete treatment with Zoloft. A switch to Prozac for those unable to tolerate Zoloft is equally effective. My colleagues and I have found that people who cannot tolerate one SSRI are often able to stand another. The minority who may feel "wired" on Prozac may feel less so on Zoloft. Prozac seems to make some people more anxious, restless, stimulated, and headachy than Zoloft. On the other hand, Zoloft may cause more hand tremors, drowsiness, diarrhea, and dry mouth. These differences are not very great, but may account for why someone could not tolerate one but could tolerate the other. When a person considers taking an SSRI, the issue of potential side effects should not guide him in his decision to take one of these agents over another. Your friend may say Prozac drove her up the wall, while Zoloft restored her health, but this report cannot help you, because your reaction may be the opposite.

Zoloft is effective in treating obsessive-compulsive disorder and all the other conditions I listed in the section on SSRIs in general, and on Prozac in particular. No SSRI has been found to be uniquely effective in treating a condition where the others are not.

Drug/Drug Interactions

Zoloft, like the other SSRIs, cannot be safely combined with an MAOI. In its favor, it, along with Celexa, has the reputation of posing less risk among the SSRIs for interactions with other drugs listed in the general section on SSRI interactions on pages 91 to 93. While this does not obviate the need for close supervision by your physician, it may allow you both to be a little less concerned.

Paxil (Paroxetine)

Paxil, the third SSRI to be released in the United States (1993), is as effective as Prozac and Zoloft, or, put less delicately, is no more curative than the others. Its sales account for almost half of the newer antidepressants sold in the United States and top $2 billion. Claims that it acts faster remain unproven. Its marketing has focused on the speed and method by which it moves through the body after ingestion (so-called pharmacokinetics). What the physician in a hurry is supposed to believe is that Paxil, unlike the others, has no active metabolites, moves through the body fastest (pharmacokinetics), and is highly serotonin-selective. Thus, the doctor is able to adjust the patient's blood level of the drug more easily and to control it best. There are several problems with this scenario. First, blood levels of all SSRIs do not correlate with cure rate or side effect incidence, and therefore no clinician measures them. Second, Paxil may have no active metabolite, but Zoloft's so-called active metabolite is not very active. And finally, physicians think that due to the long duration of Prozac in the body, it is like stopping the *Titanic* if some bad side effect occurs, but there is no actual evidence that Prozac's side effects are more sinister or long-lasting than the other SSRIs. To counteract Paxil's no-active-metabolite purity, the makers of Zoloft have charged that it mucks up the liver enzymes that break down other drugs like desipramine, as well as Paxil itself, causing the blood levels of each to rise. Again, so what? The first problem is easily dealt with by giving lower desipramine doses, and the second makes no difference, since when the blood level of Paxil rises slowly over a week, nothing bad happens. The final point of the marketing is serotonin selectivity. It used to be that Zoloft's makers could say it was more serotonin-selective than Prozac, but now Paxil is more serotonin-selective. Perhaps I am overly sensitive to advertising's attempts to influence me subconsciously, to make me feel more cultivated if I drink a certain beverage, more intelligent if I read a particular magazine, and more scientific a physician if I use the most specific of the selective serotonin reuptake inhibitors. In the back of my mind resonates nonspecific treatments that are nothing but placebos, that owe their effect to the enthusiasm and authority of the doctor rather than to the biological action of the drug itself. Doctors want, with laserlike accuracy, to kill the cancer cells and not the surrounding normal tissue, and psychiatrists want to manipulate the serotonin core of depression powerfully. Unfortunately, the serotonin levels are not the only factor to consider in comparing various drugs' efficacy. All the SSRIs are equally effective, and although on the ad scoreboard Paxil has beaten Prozac in serotonin selectivity 320 to 20, the all-around score, in fact, is tied.

Curiously, the quest for purity in serotonin selectivity has recently been replaced by dual-acting serotonin and norepinephrine antidepressants, which are deemed by the advertisers and supported to some extent by the researchers to be even more effective. In 2002 the *American Journal of Psychiatry* published a study claiming that 40 mg of Paxil also acted on norepinephrine, making it a dual-acting drug at higher doses.

Dosage

Most people can tolerate a starting dose of 20 mg of Paxil, which requires no change over the two to four weeks before the therapeutic effect begins to be felt, nor any for the whole duration on the drug. Some experience too many side effects initially and split the 20 mg tablet in half or take the 10 mg one until they get used to the side effects, and later are able to tolerate the full dosage. After a month on 20 mg, if the person has not recovered, the dose may be raised by 10 mg weekly until a daily maximum of 50 mg is reached.

Just marketed, Paxil CR is a controlled-release version available in 12.5-mg, 25-mg, and 37.5-mg tablets. It allegedly has fewer gastrointestinal side effects such as nausea (14 versus 23 percent), dry mouth, constipation, and diarrhea than does standard Paxil, and thus fewer patients drop out. Generic paroxetine is now available.

Side Effects

In addition to causing the same side effects as the other SSRIs on the gastrointestinal tract, nervous system, and sexual functions, Paxil seems more likely to cause sweating, constipation, dry mouth, drowsiness, and fatigue, and less likely to cause nervousness and diarrhea. If, for example, nervousness has been a problem on Prozac, Paxil may be a sensible second choice. The sexual difficulties caused by Paxil can be converted within days to a virtue in the treatment of premature ejaculation, without harming erectile function or libido.

The following is a story of someone who couldn't tolerate Prozac well, but was greatly helped by Paxil. John is forty-seven years old and has been very depressed since being fired from his job as an industrial engineer. He knows he should be mailing out résumés and networking with colleagues, but cannot get himself to do either. John has trouble falling and staying asleep, feels slowed down and without energy, and is convinced no one will hire him. He has black circles around his eyes; he barely speaks to his wife and snaps at his children. John cannot concentrate on anything he tries to read or write, and worries constantly about the future. After months of suffering, he took a friend's recommendation and came to see me. I started him on Prozac, and we began to talk about his illness and his life. After several weeks, he told me he could not stand the drug, that he was now up all night worrying and frightened, and that he felt tense and unable to relax. The anxiety of most depressed people is diminished by Prozac, but about 10 percent grow more upset from it, and become worse than before. John belonged to this minority.

I suggested he stop taking Prozac, wait a few days, and then begin half the normal 20-mg Paxil dose (the tablet is scored and easily divided). The reason for the lower dose is that Prozac would leave his system very slowly, and I did not want to wait until it was completely gone because of his suffering. Starting him on 10 mg of Paxil would be safe, and in a week I raised it to 20 mg. Two weeks later, he began to feel more energetic, to sleep better, and to make necessary phone calls. In a month, he was singing the praises of Paxil, as he actively pursued his job search.

The Properties of Paxil

Like Prozac and Zoloft, Paxil is safe and effective in the moderately to severely depressed, the anxious depressed, and the elderly. Since half of major depressives relapse in two years, and 80 to 90 percent who have suffered two episodes go on to have a third, prevention of further outbreaks of the illness is essential. Paxil, like the other SSRIs, decreases the relapse rate by about 30 percent.

Paxil is like Prozac in its blocking the liver enzyme metabolism of itself and other drugs, and like Zoloft in being shorter-acting. Its absorption is not affected by food or antacids. Except for the elderly and those with liver or kidney damage, who require lower amounts, most people start out on 20 mg in the morning and stay on it until recovery.

Paxil normalizes the sleep patterns in depressed people, unlike Prozac and Luvox, and helps those who take it in the morning to fall asleep at night and feel more rested the next day. In spite of this, the degree of insomnia as a side effect of all SSRIs is about the same. Like Prozac, Paxil does not increase the drive toward suicide. In fact, they both lessen it.

If a patient has been on Paxil for months or more, suddenly discontinuing use of it is (of the SSRIs) most likely to cause very unpleasant withdrawal symptoms. These range from some odd and terrifying headaches and "brain shocks" to fatigue and/or insomnia. Flulike symptoms of running nose, sweating, nausea, vomiting, diarrhea, and muscle pain may occur. Sometimes a migraine-like illness evolves, accompanied by severe dizziness and the seeing of small floating shapes. It is believed that Paxil is more likely to produce unpleasant withdrawal effects because of its shorter duration of action (it has a twenty-four-hour half-life) and lack of active metabolites. These are least likely to occur if the patient has taken Prozac, which is eliminated very slowly. Physical withdrawal symptoms have been reported to arise even when the dose of Paxil is tapered off very slowly over a week or two.

Dizziness is the most common SSRI withdrawal symptom, often accompanied by blurred vision. The second most common is the sensation of tingling and burning. Withdrawal symptoms begin two to five days after the SSRI is stopped. Paxil and Luvox are the most likely to cause withdrawal reactions, with Zoloft and Celexa less so. Prozac is the least likely to cause them, but definitely can do so. Effexor also can produce withdrawal reactions, while Serzone does not seem to do so.

Drug/Drug Interactions

There are three levels of drug interactions with Paxil, as there are with Prozac and to a lesser extent with Zoloft and Celexa: (1) the severe, (2) the moderate, and (3) the mild. The severe interactions involve the MAOIs Nardil and Parnate and any other drug that raises the level of serotonin, like tryptophan. The moderate interactions involve combinations with other drugs whose levels in the body are raised much higher than one might otherwise suspect. For example, if the normal dose of approximately 250 mg of desipramine were administered with Paxil or Prozac, it would be like giving 1,000 mg of the drug, which could cause serious toxicity. As mentioned earlier, an easy way around this problem is to give 50 mg of desipramine to people taking Paxil. This caution applies to other tricyclics and antipsychotics, like molindone.

The list of mild interactions is longest and constantly being added to. It includes those for all SSRIs, noted on pages 91 to 93, such as the increased danger of bleeding when on an anticoagulant, and the need for caution when taking antihistamines, anticonvulsants, antiarrhythmics, beta-blockers, and various psychiatric drugs. Remember to be careful when combining medications, and always consult your doctor before doing so.

Summary

Paxil is a safe and effective SSRI. It has the usual SSRI side effects on the gastrointestinal tract, the nervous system, and on sexual functioning. But it also shares the advantages of the SSRIs: (1) dosing is easy (one pill daily), (2) it is reasonably well tolerated, (3) it has no effect on the heart or blood pressure, (4) it has no effect on a person's ability to drive a car or other motor skills, and (5) there are few serious drug/drug interactions.

Luvox (Fluvoxamine)

In 1995, the Food and Drug Administration approved Luvox, which has been prescribed in Switzerland since 1983, five years before Prozac was released in the United States. The drug is used to treat depression in Europe, but is approved in the United States only for obsessive-compulsive disorder (OCD). Nonetheless, any physician who wishes to prescribe it for depression can do so legally. In spite of the fact that Solvay, the European manufacturer of Luvox, asserts that 37,000 patients have been studied in controlled clinical trials and that by 1992 4.5 million had been treated with the drug, there remains some doubt about the antidepressant efficacy of Luvox, because some of the small placebo-controlled studies found it positive and others negative. Thus, Solvay and Upjohn, the American manufacturer of Luvox, have the third approved medication for OCD following the tricyclic Anafranil, and the SSRI Prozac, but their application for its use as an antidepressant is still being reviewed by the FDA. The attempt to establish Luvox as OCD-specific seems mainly a marketing ploy, since all SSRIs are effective for OCD and depression. To my knowledge, no comparative studies have established Luvox as superior to the other SSRIs for OCD.

In addition to OCD, Luvox will undoubtedly be used to treat other repetitive behaviors (e.g., voyeurism, other sexual perversions and addictions, and behaviors exhibited by the autistic child). It will also be prescribed, as have other SSRIs, for Tourette's syndrome (characterized by tics, grunts, and obscenities), body dysmorphic disorders (feeling ugly or deformed although normal-looking), binge eating, self-injurious behavior, and pathologic jealousy.

Characteristics of Luvox

Its absorption is not affected by food. Half a dose of Luvox is eliminated by the body in fifteen hours, and it has no active metabolites (drug breakdown products). The dose range is 50 to 300 mg daily, and the manufacturer recommends that amounts above 100 mg be given in divided doses, with the larger one taken at bedtime. Presumably, this is because of the drug's rapid metabolism and perhaps also because nausea, which occurs in 40 percent of cases, will be lessened by not taking all the drug at once. The 50- and 100-mg tablets are scored for easy division. Luvox comes in 25-, 50-, and 100-mg sizes. The need to take it twice a day is a disadvantage of Luvox versus the other SSRIs. Also, since the treatment of OCD by SSRIs typically requires higher doses than those needed for depression, Luvox's nausea problem could be significant. I have never found any need to prescribe this drug, nor have I ever noticed it on any list of best-sellers.

Side Effects

Luvox's side effects are typical of an SSRI: nausea, dyspepsia, abdominal pain, vomiting, sexual dysfunction, sleepiness, insomnia, nervousness, weakness, dizziness, constipation, and diarrhea. The drug usually does not cause weight gain, and is comparatively safe in overdose. Details of how its side effects compare with those of the other SSRIs have yet to be revealed. Like Paxil, with no active metabolites and a shorter half-life, it is more likely to cause a withdrawal syndrome if its use is suddenly discontinued.

Drug/Drug Interactions

Luvox interacts with tricyclic antidepressants, Coumadin (it raises the blood level of this anticoagulant, increasing the chance of bleeding), Tegretol, Dilantin, Inderal, methadone, and Valium (take Ativan instead). The drug does not seem to interact with the heart medicine digoxin, or with alcohol. Luvox cannot be given within two weeks of MAOIs like Nardil or Parnate. There can be danger to the heart in combining Luvox with the antihistamines Seldane and Hismanal and the antifungal agent Nizoral. Seldane and Hismanal have been withdrawn from the market.

Luvox and Other Drugs in Obsessive-Compulsive Disorder (OCD)

As mentioned earlier, obsessions are unwanted, usually horrific thoughts, impulses, and images that are experienced by the sufferer as products of his own mind which are inappropriate and should be suppressed, and that cause anxiety. Behavioral and mental compulsions include hand-washing, arranging and checking (e.g., is the gas off?) behaviors, and mental acts (e.g., counting, endlessly reviewing conversations for hidden meaning), useless repetitions that a person is driven to perform to decrease stress or magically prevent a dreaded event. These obsessions and compulsions cause marked distress, are time-consuming (more than an hour a day), or interfere with social or occupational functioning.

The word *compulsive* is used in everyday parlance to refer to excessive eating, drinking, sex, and gambling, but these activities are experienced as pleasurable, whereas true compulsions are not. Unlike the obsessive-compulsive personality (OCP), who is proud of his orderliness, punctuality, and frugality, the OCD experiences his thoughts and impulses as disgusting, horrific, and to be controlled.

On April 25, 1994, Michael Miller, writing in the *Wall Street Journal*, warned of an advertising plot by "two giant companies, Upjohn and Solvay," makers of Luvox, to reach the large numbers of OCD sufferers who go undiagnosed and untreated in order to increase sale of this drug. The author speaks of the packaging and marketing of diseases to people. These two companies spent $1 million, Miller reported, to hire a public relations firm to promote a slogan about "unlocking the Captive Mind" to doctors, patients, and their families. They also funded Dr. Robert DuPont, Miller continues, to study the annual economic costs of OCD, and the preliminary conclusion was between $8 and $10 billion. Next, Miller noted that another psychiatrist, Wayne Goodman of the University of Florida, was preparing a short quiz for consumers to determine if they have signs of OCD. A strategy like this will most likely work, if the experience with attention deficit hyperactivity disorder (ADHD) is any guide. I answered a questionnaire in *The New York Times Book Review* advertising a popular book on the subject, and found I had seventeen positive signs for the disorder out of twenty. It is no accident that sales of Ritalin, used to treat this condition, have sharply increased in the past year. I do not mean to imply that ADHD is not real, any more than OCD is not one of the most painful illnesses imaginable. I am referring instead to the practice of marketing the mildest forms of these conditions to the public. Upjohn and Solvay are now looking for a celebrity sufferer of OCD to advertise it. Perhaps their difficulty in finding one means that the true disorder is rare after all, and that if a person really had it, he would be socially isolated, celibate, and spending days in meaningless activities, rather than famous.

If you nonetheless decide to try Luvox, give it three months to work. About one third to half of those on it improve. Those who get better need to keep taking the drug or they will relapse, and they tend not to get completely well. For those who do not completely recover, the best therapy (in addition to the drug) is behavioral therapy, which directly exposes them to the terrifying dirt or germ, prevents them from washing, and teaches them to control their anxiety and calm themselves. Confronting pictures of or imagining the terrifying situation does not work as well as real contact.

If a person with OCD decides to try Paxil, 40 to 60 mg works better than the usual 20-mg dose. For Zoloft, a maximum dose of 200 mg may be necessary. Higher doses of Prozac (40 to 80 mg) also seem to be more effective than the standard 20 mg. High-dose Celexa and Lexapro are also effective. Occasionally, a person will do better on a lower than usual SSRI dosage. If an OCD sufferer also has tics (blinking, shoulder-shrugging, throat-clearing), a low dose of an antipsychotic drug like Haldol added to Luvox can be helpful.

Summary

Luvox is an old drug, introduced in 1995 to America, and in 1983 to Europe. Its drawbacks are that it must be used twice daily (instead of once) because of its rapid metabolism, and there is some question about its effectiveness in treating depression. Marketed specifically for OCD, I would applaud a more powerful action in OCD than that of the tricyclic Ana-franil or the other SSRIs, but so far there is no evidence of this. As a psychiatrist, I do not plan to prescribe it until its superiority for OCD is established.

Celexa (Citalopram)

In 1998, Celexa, the fifth SSRI, was approved for release in the United States for the treatment of depression, although it had been widely used in Europe since 1989, which, like Luvox, makes it a new old drug. Having been given to over 20,000 subjects in clinical trials, and used by over 20 million people worldwide, the drug is safe and effective. It may become eligible for generic release as early as 2004.

Characteristics of Celexa

Half eliminated by the body in thirty-five hours, its usual dose range is 10 to 60 mg taken once daily. Absorption is not affected by food. The drug is available in 10-, 20-, and 40-mg scored tablets. Some people feel better starting on 10 mg a day for several days. In Europe, as much as 80 mg a day has been prescribed. The 40-mg dose may be more effective than the 20-mg. A liquid form (10mg/5ml) also is available.

Side Effects

These are comparable to other SSRIs and include nausea, dry mouth, sleepiness, and delayed ejaculation. Celexa is slightly sedating rather than activating. The drug is secreted in human breast milk. Large overdoses of Celexa have slowed conduction in the heart, caused convulsions, and resulted in twelve deaths from the drug in combination with other medications and two from Celexa alone.

Drug/Drug Interactions

Like other SSRIs, it should not be combined with MAOIs. It seems to have less influence on liver metabolism than other SSRIs and therefore may cause fewer drug-interaction difficulties. This may be of special value to elderly patients on many medications.

Summary

Celexa is equal to the other SSRIs in therapeutic efficacy for the treatment of depression and probably also for obsessive-compulsive disorder and panic disorder. Its minimal effect on liver metabolism, and thereby interactions with other medical and psychiatric drugs, makes it attractive in the treatment of the elderly, medically ill, and those on other psychiatric medications.

Lexapro (Escitalopram)

In 2002, Lexapro (escitalopram), a new SSRI, was approved by the FDA, raising expectations in those for whom previous antidepressants had either been ineffective or produced unbearable side effects. Since 30 percent of those who have tried medications had not been helped, and many others could not stand the gastrointestinal, sleep, and sexual disturbances, plus the fatigue and drugged feeling caused by them, Lexapro excites new hope. Many physicians are eager to prescribe it, and their patients to take it.

Lexapro is a purified version of Celexa. To explain the method of producing it will introduce you to more chemistry than you want to know. Briefly, it is an isomer that is the same compound as Celexa, but differs in the position of the atoms in the molecule, and presumably is more efficient at the synapse in its effect, and less likely to produce side effects. The old Celexa was a mixture of L- and R-citalopram. The new Lexapro eliminates the R-citalopram, which presumably had been responsible for side effects and caused a drag on clinical effectiveness.

Characteristics of Lexapro

With a half-life of twenty-seven to thirty-two hours, and once-daily dosing with 10- and 20-mg scored (easily breakable) tablets, 10 mg per day of Lexapro compares to 40 mg per day of Celexa, and is usually enough.

Presumed Advantages

One claim made for Lexapro over Celexa is more rapid onset of action. Its effect is statistically significant after only one week, whereas it takes four to six weeks for Celexa (see figure and table below). If this finding holds up in subsequent studies, and if it is clinically, not just statistically significant, of which I am afraid I am doubtful (look again at Gorman's data), then it will be an important contribution.

Mean Change from Baseline in MADRS Scores

Mean change from baseline in MADRS total score in placebo-, citalopram-, and escitalopram-treated patients. Represented are OC values by visit (weeks 1–8), and LOCF values at end point (week 8).

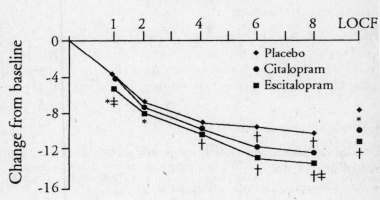

Treatment week

*$P < .05$ versus placebo.
†$P < .001$ versus placebo.
‡$P < .05$ escitalopram versus citalopram.
MADRS = Montgomery Asberg Depression Rating Scale;
OC = observed cases; LOCF = last observation carried forward.
Gorman, J.M. Korotzer, A. Su, G. *CNS Spectrums*. Vol. 7, No. 4 (suppl. 1), 2002.

LOCF Values by Visit for the Major Efficacy Parameters, MADRS, and CGI-I

Study Week	Placebo	Escitalopram	Citalopram
MADRS			
1	−3.8	−4.7*,†	−3.7
2	−6.6	−7.8*	−7.2
4	−9.4	−11.0*	−10.2

Study Week	Placebo	Escitalopram	Citalopram
6	−10.3	−13.0*,†	−12.0*
8	−11.2	−13.8*	−13.1*
MADRS severe			
1	−4.2	−5.5*,†	−4.3
2	−7.4	−9.0*	−7.9
4	−10.4	−12.2*	−11.3
6	−11.7	−14.7*,†	−12.8*
8	−12.2	−16.2*,†	−14.3*
CGI-I			
1	3.5	3.3*	3.4
2	3.2	3.0*	3.1
4	2.9	2.6*	2.7*
6	2.8	2.4*	2.5*
8	2.7	2.4*	2.3*

Shown are the mean changes from baseline in MADRS total score for the entire pooled population (MADRS), and for the subset that were severely depressed at baseline (MADRS severe; baseline MADRS ≥ 30), as well as the mean CG1-I scores for the entire pooled population.
*$P < .05$ for active treatment versus placebo.
†$P < .05$ escitalopram versus citalopram.
Gorman, J.M. Korotzer, A. Su, G. *CNS Spectrums*. Vol. 7, No. 4 (suppl. 1), 2002.

One of the great problems when a person is in severe pain from depression is how slowly the antidepressants work. Many, over the last twenty-five or more years, have promised faster results, only to not deliver. If Lexapro, in fact, does, it is a significant advance. The drug must stand up to the clinician's and patient's ongoing scrutiny now that it has passed that of the FDA.

Side Effects

The most common side effects are insomnia and nausea. Lexapro has been found to have several advantages over Celexa (see table below).

Most Common Adverse Events Reported in Escitalopram (Lexapro) and Citalopram (Celexa)

	Placebo (n = 1,038)	Lexapro (n = 715)	Celexa (n = 1,471)
Nausea	10%	15%	20%
Insomnia	8%	9%	13%
Dry mouth	9%	6%	17%
Somnolence	5%	6%	14%
Diarrhea	5%	8%	9%
Dizziness	6%	5%	9%
Sweating	5%	5%	9%

Owens, M.J., Rosenbaum, J.F. *CNS Spectrums.* Vol. 7, No. 4 (suppl. 1), 2002.

Drug/Drug Interactions

Do not combine Lexapro with MAOIs. There is minimal effect on liver metabolism compared to other SSRIs with fewer interaction problems, making Lexapro a candidate for use in the elderly or medically ill who are on many other drugs, and for those on psychiatric medications.

Summary

Lexapro has the right credentials to pass through the scrutiny of the FDA, and there is no reason to believe it will not prove to be safe and effective. But now we need the years of experience with it in normal clinical practice to discover its true nature. If it lives up to its promise of faster action and fewer side effects, it will prove a welcome addition. If not, the wait will continue for the next drug or a new answer.

Are There Any Differences in Side Effects Among the SSRIs?

In large studies, statistically significant differences among the SSRIs are difficult to show, and the drugs seem very much alike. Paxil causes the least diarrhea and most constipation and therefore, if a person cannot tolerate the loose stools caused by Prozac, Zoloft, or Celexa, Paxil is a reasonable alternative. If the dry mouth caused by Zoloft, Paxil, or Celexa is a problem, perhaps a change to Prozac or Lexapro would help. Zoloft, Paxil, Celexa, and Lexapro probably cause less nervousness than Prozac, but Paxil and Celexa may cause more fatigue and drowsiness. If you are wired from Prozac, try Paxil, Celexa, or Lexapro; if you are sluggish from Paxil, try Prozac.

I have constructed a table comparing the side effects of the five drugs based on averages from a number of studies. Most of the adverse reactions occur less than 10 percent of the time, and many of them are minor and disappear in a few weeks. The table is based on a system of one to three plus signs, with one being the least likelihood of a side effect, and three being the most.

Possible Side Effect Differences Among the SSRIs

	Prozac	Zoloft	Paxil	Celexa	Lexapro
Nervousness/insomnia	++	+	+	+	+
Drowsiness and fatigue	+	+	++	++	+
Dry mouth	+	++	++	+++	+
Weight gain	+	+	+	+	?
Diarrhea	+	++	+	++	++
Sweating	+	+	++	++	+

Key
+++ = high
  ++ = notable
    + = low

It has been my experience that Prozac and Paxil are the most dissimilar in terms of the side effects they produce, and Celexa has the fewest interactions with other drugs.

SSRI Summary

There are three reasons why the SSRIs as a class are now the most widely prescribed antidepressants: the ease of taking them, their tolerability, and their safety in overdose.

Dosage

The once-daily starting dose is usually also the maximum dose. Gone is the need, in most instances, to gradually elevate drug intake from one to twelve tablets a day, as with the tricyclic antidepressants.

Tolerability

Although 20 percent of people who start on an SSRI stop taking it within weeks, and another 15 percent within months, because of side effects, the large majority suffer little or no discomfort from them. These drugs do not interfere with driving and other skilled tasks, and do not increase the effects of alcohol. Thus, more people complete the treatment at full dosage for an acute depressive episode, and those who need to are able to continue long-term therapy to prevent relapse. The gastrointestinal side effects, at first troubling to some, usually can be tolerated and eventually subside, as do the side effects on the central nervous system, such as anxiety and sleep disturbance. Unfortunately, the sexual difficulties induced by the SSRIs are fairly common, occurring in 30 to 50 or more percent by some estimates, and for many physicians and patients constitute the prime weakness of these agents. The list of rare side effects and drug/drug interactions is growing, as more experience with these medications is gathered, making it essential that you keep in touch with your prescribing physician.

Safety in Overdose

The illness of depression is often accompanied by suicidal thoughts and impulses, as well as actual suicide attempts. The SSRIs are fairly safe in overdose, which allows the doctor to prescribe adequate amounts without excessive fear. The danger of suicide with tricyclic antidepressants is one of the reasons they were given in too small doses, and thus did not produce a full therapeutic effect.

SSRIs, in spite of an early erroneous report and recent concerns about children, do not increase suicidal ideas, impulses, and actions. In overdose, they usually do not affect the heart, pulse rate, or blood pressure, nor do they cause any severe nervous system response (e.g., seizure, coma), and as a result, very few deaths from SSRI overdose occur.

If Prozac, Zoloft, Paxil, Luvox, Celexa, and Lexapro are so good, why are there three more chapters in this book describing even more antidepressants? The answer has to do with efficacy and side effects. About 30 percent of the people who try them do not respond to SSRIs, and perhaps another 20 percent are improved, but not completely cured. Furthermore, the rate of response and cure is too slow, so that the search for faster relief must continue. And finally, the SSRIs are not tolerated by everyone (perhaps 35 percent), the main reason being the sexual side effects.

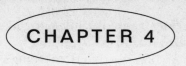

CHAPTER 4

The New Antidepressants: Wellbutrin, Effexor, Serzone, Remeron, and Cymbalta (Duloxetine)

There are four other new antidepressants that are currently available—Wellbutrin, Effexor, Serzone, and Remeron—and one that very soon will be, Cymbalta (duloxetine). New drugs are like new cars; they look good, but no one knows how they will wear. Wellbutrin was subject to a recall by its manufacturer weeks after its initial release in 1986, and its image has still not completely recovered although it has fewer sexual side effects. Effexor requires the dose to be individually tailored, unlike the once-a-day SSRIs, and blood pressure must be monitored regularly in order to detect the hypertension the drug sometimes causes. Serzone causes less insomnia, anxiety, and sexual dysfunction, but its rare liver toxicity has resulted in its being withdrawn in Europe and Canada. Remeron may be calming and may cause fewer sexual side effects, but it also may make too many feel drugged and fatigued, gain weight, and have their white blood cell count threatened. Cymbalta, a soon-to-be-released dual (serotonin *and* norepinephrine) reuptake inhibitor like Effexor, will be marketed as more likely to completely cure rather than merely improve depression, and to relieve pain in various parts of the body, such as the back.

The ongoing appetite for new antidepressants exists because of the failures of the old ones. While the majority of people taking them have been helped, 30 percent do not respond, and an additional 20 percent are not completely cured. Also, the episodic nature of depression allows the sufferer to take a new drug after a new occurrence. Side effects cause 20 percent to go off the first antidepressant soon after starting, and an additional 15 percent to discontinue it within a year. It is estimated that if you are depressed, your first medication will fail you about 40 percent of the time, either because it does not work or because it makes you too uncomfortable. This leaves the market wide open for agents that are presumably more effective or better tolerated. It is good to have Wellbutrin, Effexor, Serzone, Remeron, and Cymbalta as alternatives for those who have not been helped by or cannot tolerate the SSRIs.

Wellbutrin

Wellbutrin was about to be released in 1986, two years before Prozac, as an effective antidepressant with the same advantages over tricyclics as the SSRIs—namely, less dry mouth, blurred vision, constipation, weight gain, drop in blood pressure, or danger to the heart. In a 1986 prerelease study, the drug caused four grand mal seizures in 55 nondepressed bulimic women, and it was withdrawn for further testing. Burroughs Wellcome, the manufacturer of Wellbutrin, went on to study the frequency of Wellbutrin-induced seizures in 3,000 depressed patients, and found that if it was given in a maximum amount of 150 mg three times a day up to 450 mg total daily, the seizure rate was roughly comparable to that with other antidepressants. The reason for the 150-mg ceiling for a given amount is that seizures are significantly dose-related, and most likely to occur after a given dose or dose change. Missed portions should not be "doubled up" next time the drug is taken. At 1 in 250, the seizure rate was about the same as with the tricyclics. The seizure rate for all patients on Prozac in a similar premarketing study was 1 in 500, which is not very different, while that for Zoloft and Paxil was less than 1 in 1,000. Seizures in tricyclics occur in 1 out of 200 patients taking average doses of 150 mg a day. The incidence of seizures in a survey of patients not on antidepressants in general practice in Britain was 0.4 percent, or the same 1 in 250 as that found for Wellbutrin. It has been concluded that seizures are unlikely to occur if Wellbutrin is given in divided doses of less than 150 mg at a time to people who are *not* bulimic and do not possess other predisposing factors for seizures, such as a history of epilepsy, alcoholism, head trauma, brain tumor, fever, or drugs lowering the seizure threshold (e.g., tricyclics, antipsychotics, lithium, short-acting benzodiazepines like Halcion and Xanax). The drug was rereleased three years later, in 1989. But the seizure history limited its use until only recently, when it was found that those who take it are unlikely to experience drug-related impairment of their sexual functioning. Maybe it was more acceptable than the SSRIs after all. Nonetheless, the need to raise the dose slowly and to take as many as nine pills daily in three divided doses made it cumbersome to use. To overcome this handicap, the manufacturer has issued a sustained release form of the drug (Wellbutrin SR) that can be taken up to a maximum of 200 mg twice daily. The necessity of gradually elevating the dose would remain, but would be simpler on a twice-daily basis. Wellbutrin SR comes in 100- and 150-mg tablets. Wellbutrin XL (150 mg and 300 mg) has just been released and is taken only once a day.

How Wellbutrin actually works is unknown. It has no effect on serotonin and only modest effects on norepinephrine and dopamine. This makes it different from all other antidepressants in use, and makes it desirable, perhaps, for people who are not helped by other drugs.

The Effectiveness of Wellbutrin

Wellbutrin is no more curative than other new antidepressants and has been well studied. Although it is an activating drug like Prozac, it also reduces anxiety, even in those depressed patients who are anxious before treatment. It can be safely taken by people with heart disease, high blood pressure, and other illnesses. In depressives who neither respond to nor can tolerate other drugs, Wellbutrin has been effective in from a half to two thirds of cases. It has been found effective in people who don't respond to the tricyclics. Patients who have suffered sexual side effects on SSRIs often do well on Wellbutrin. Sporadic studies, in need of controlled confirmation, suggest that Wellbutrin does not destabilize the moods of bipolar depressives, as do other antidepressants, tipping fewer into mania or rapid cycling (more than four manic or depressive episodes per year). The drug has also been used (but is not FDA-approved) to effectively treat chronic fatigue syndrome. It is said *not* to be effective in treating depression associated with panic disorder, in pure panic disorder, or in obsessive-compulsive disorder. In fact, Wellbutrin is the only antidepressant apparently not useful in the treatment of anxiety disorders. The drug seems to be too stimulating for anxious patients. Nonetheless, there was a study comparing Wellbutrin SR and Zoloft that found them equally effective in the treatment of anxiety.

One bright example of a case in which Wellbutrin worked where eight other antidepressants had failed is a forty-four-year-old patient of mine. Bob had suffered six-month-long major depressive episodes every two years since his late teens. Although he had never been hospitalized, they succeeded in destroying his life, interrupting his education so that it took ten years for him to complete his course in accounting, and ruined all his jobs. Although he finally completed his course work, he had not been able to pass his certified public accounting test and was working part time as a bartender. The ten major depressive episodes that came over him without apparent cause had resulted in his losing track of most of his friends, and all but a few family members. When he was ill, he had no appetite, could not sleep, would burst into tears without cause, was unable to concentrate on what he read, and had no energy to work. The fact that at those times his sex drive was zero seemed minor. He had been treated without much success with five tricyclic antidepressants (Elavil, Tofranil, desipramine, Pamelor, and Sinequan) as well as three different SSRIs (Prozac, Zoloft, and Paxil). Not only had they failed him in the acute phase, they had not been able to prevent his biannual recurrences. Wellbutrin not only sped recovery from his eleventh episode, it prevented relapse for seven years. Although it is too early to pronounce him cured forever, the drug has spared him long enough so far that he has been able to get a better job, save money, get married, and buy a home. For Bob, Wellbutrin has worked a minor miracle.

Dosage

One hundred milligrams of Wellbutrin is taken in the morning and evening for the first three days, and on the fourth, a midday 100-mg tablet is added. If a dose is forgotten, it cannot be corrected by doubling the next amount because of the danger of seizure induction. The maximum dosage for those not responsive to less is 150 mg for the immediate-release formulation three times a day, although 300 mg is usually enough.

Zyban (bupropion HCL) is a slow-release form of Wellbutrin that has been approved by the FDA to aid in giving up smoking. The drug is started a week before a person tries to stop. The most common side effects are headache, sleeplessness, and dry mouth. A dosage of 150 mg twice a day is the most effective course in helping people end smoking and avoid subsequent weight gain. After a year twice as many who took Zyban as opposed to placebo remained nonsmokers, but, unfortunately, three quarters of the Zyban group were smoking again. Wellbutrin SR, available in 100- and 150-mg tablets, is exactly the same as Zyban, and is taken twice daily to a maximum of 400 mg per day. No single dose of the sustained-release formulation should exceed 200 mg. Since Wellbutrin is broken down by the body into several amphetamine-like compounds, it is commonly used as an effective substitute for stimulants in the treatment of attention deficit/hyperactivity disorder in children and adults.

Side Effects

When it was originally released in 1986, two years before Prozac, Wellbutrin was set to be the best antidepressant because it produced the fewest side effects. It had the tricyclics beat because it caused less or no sedation, postural hypotension, dry mouth, sweating, blurred vision, constipation, weight gain, sexual dysfunction, rapid pulse, urinary retention, enhancement of alcohol or other central nervous system depressants, and disturbances of memory. But because the release of Wellbutrin was delayed for three years due to its seizure problem, it was not available in 1988 when Prozac was released, offering *almost* the same list of benefits. Prozac quickly became number one in the nation and the world. Wellbutrin is now, as I noted earlier, making a modest comeback against Prozac because of its much lower incidence of sexual side effects. Neither Wellbutrin nor the SSRIs adversely affect the heart, and both are safe in overdose.

The most common side effects of Wellbutrin are gastrointestinal and stimulatory, just as with Prozac. Patients may suffer nausea and mild dry mouth, but those who cannot tolerate Wellbutrin usually cannot because of its stimulatory effects, which they find unbearable. Agitation, insomnia, anxiety, and tremors are the reasons for the rare premature discontinuation of treatment. Most often the stimulatory effects occur early in treatment, soon gradually subside, and are less of a problem if the dose is low at first and very slowly raised. Because of its stimulatory effects, Wellbutrin should not be taken at bedtime. Sleep disturbance due to depression responds slowly to Wellbutrin, because all antidepressants take weeks to act, and a sleeping pill may be necessary at the beginning of treatment. In 5 to 10 percent of the women who take it, Wellbutrin can disrupt menstruation.

Wellbutrin's Lower Incidence of Sexual Dysfunction

Estimates of sexual dysfunction on Prozac range from 2 to 75 percent. In a study of thirty-one patients who had had difficulty with orgasm on Prozac and who were taken off all psychiatric medications for two weeks and then put on Wellbutrin for at least four weeks, 84 percent reported improved orgasm, more sexual satisfaction, and increased desire. Wellbutrin never worsened orgasmic function. Its most common side effects were anxiety, agitation, nausea, constipation, and headaches. Because this study was not blinded (both the patients and the doctors knew the treatment being given), the patients' expectations may have influenced the outcome. Nonetheless, it seems to support the notion that Wellbutrin does not interfere with sexual functioning. Another pair of researchers (E. A. Gardner and J. A. Johnston) found that diminished sexual desire resulting from antidepressants went away when Wellbutrin was substituted. Diminished sexual desire is often caused by depression as well as the drug treating it, whereas inhibition or absence of ejaculation or of orgasm is due not to the illness but to the antidepressant drug. While Wellbutrin improves or does not harm all of these sexual functions, its effect on desire is harder to determine. There have been reported cases in which antidepressant-caused sexual dysfunction by Effexor or an SSRI was relieved by the addition of 75 to 150 mg of Wellbutrin.

Overdose

Overdose deaths from Wellbutrin alone are extremely rare. About one third of those who overdose develop seizures but recover. Rapid heartbeat and hypotension also occur. Wellbutrin overdoses must be carefully treated.

Side Effects Compared to the SSRIs

The nonsexual side effect frequency due to Wellbutrin is low, and there are few significant differences between Wellbutrin and the SSRIs. Wellbutrin causes more nervousness and palpitations, and less fatigue, while the SSRIs cause more nausea and diarrhea. Wellbutrin causes more dry mouth and constipation, but these are usually mild. Weakness is more common with the SSRIs. The side effect differences between the drugs have not yet been carefully compared in a double-blind study.

Drug/Drug Interactions

In general, Wellbutrin's drug/drug interactions are minimal. MAOIs (Nardil, Parnate) are absolutely not to be taken with Wellbutrin. Its combination with the Parkinson's disease drug levodopa should be cautious, because of stimulatory and gastrointestinal side effects. Wellbutrin should be used with great caution or not at all with drugs that lower the seizure threshold (e.g., other antidepressants, clozapine, alcohol, short-acting benzodiazepines such as Xanax). Because of Wellbutrin's narrow dose range (below 225 mg, it has no effect, and above 450 mg, there is a danger of convulsions), other drugs that raise or lower its blood level can be dangerous. Thus, if you have been taking Prozac and want to switch, remember that Prozac leaves the body slowly and raises the level of Wellbutrin. Thus, you should wait two weeks before starting to take Wellbutrin. It is safe to give Wellbutrin with clonidine, antiarrhythmic drugs, Coumadin, and digitalis.

Summary

The sales of Wellbutrin have been growing, but continue to lag far behind those of the SSRIs. The reasons for this discrepancy lie not in the drugs' effectiveness or side-effect patterns, which are commendable, but in fear of Wellbutrin-induced seizures and the need to take even the long-acting form of the drug twice a day. When Wellbutrin is taken at the clinically effective dose of no more than 450 mg a day, its seizure rate is 4 in 1,000, quite similar to the 2 in 1,000 of Prozac, and the 3 in 1,000 of Paxil. Wellbutrin is a safe and effective antidepressant, giving people the choice between the convenient, once-daily dosage offered by the SSRIs, accompanied by a high incidence of sexual dysfunction, and a less convenient, twice-daily dosage with few sexual side effects. The new Wellbutrin XL, taken once a day, may eliminate this last objection.

Effexor

In 1994, Effexor was introduced by Wyeth-Ayerst as "Prozac with a punch," because of its action not only as an SSRI but also as a norepinephrine reuptake inhibitor (NERI), giving it a double-barreled impact on depression. The manufacturer presented it as having few side effects, like the SSRIs, accompanied by greater efficacy.

Effexor's Effectiveness

Some studies have shown that Effexor is faster-acting and more effective than Prozac and the other new antidepressants, but there is much skepticism about these claims. Over the last forty years, several antidepressant drugs have initially promised quicker relief, only to later fail to provide it. The search for relief in a matter of days rather than weeks or months is fueled by not only the suffering of patients and their families from this painful illness, but also the suicide rate of 15 percent among depressives. In prerelease studies of Effexor, the rate at which the dose was raised was faster than would be likely in normal clinical practice. This causes a faster response to the drug, but also more side effects.

Effexor is said to be more effective than other new anti-depressants in hospitalized depressives. In one recent study, it was found to be better than Prozac in the treatment of severely depressed inpatients, but more studies are necessary before it can be said with confidence that Effexor is truly more pow-erful in this group of patients. This power, if it exists, may be due to the physician's willingness to push doses higher and monitor blood pressure readings more closely in the hospital than is practical with people outside it. Thus, while Effexor's superiority to the SSRIs is an interesting point (if true), it may have little relevance for the average depressed outpatient. But if a person is suffering from a severe, otherwise unresponsive depression, then careful dose elevation to 375 mg per day, coupled with a willingness to carefully watch blood pressure and tolerate possible nausea, anxiety, insomnia, and sexual side effects, may yield the relief not available from other anti-depressants.

It is believed that Effexor initially acts primarily as an SSRI, and that its norepinephrine effect occurs at higher doses. This explains the responsiveness at higher amounts of those not helped at lesser ones.

The Effexor believers regard the drug as faster-acting, more effective in the severely ill inpatient, and able to help a third or more of those refractory to other drugs and treat-ment. While there are scraps of evidence to back all this up, they are extremely meager. The skeptics are quick to point out marketing tricks, such as comparing a new drug like Effexor with the old tricyclics at inadequate doses, so that the new agent will appear more effective, and the practice of comparing it to tricyclics with more side effects (e.g., Elavil and Tofranil) rather than to those with fewer (e.g., desipra-mine, Pamelor), so that the new agent will appear less toxic. Remember: for a drug to be released, all it need do is be more effective than a placebo and neither kill anyone nor cause other unacceptable toxicity. Comparing it in detail with existing drugs in its class comes much later, if ever. I hope Effexor is better, as its advocates claim. There clearly is a need for it.

Dosage

Unlike the SSRIs, the higher the dose of Effexor the more likely the individual will respond. This need to adjust dosage makes it more cumbersome to use. Effexor is started at 37.5 mg once or twice a day and taken with food, then moved up every four days until a total of 150 mg is reached. When necessary, the amount can be gradually raised further every four days to 225 mg per day, taken in two or three divided doses. For severely depressed patients, 350 mg daily is sometimes prescribed. It is supplied in 25-, 37.5-, 50-, 75-, and 100-mg tablets. It is half eliminated in five to eleven hours, which means twice-daily dosage is required unless the extended-release form is taken.

Effexor XR

Available in 37.5-, 75-, and 150-mg size, these extended-release capsules have been available since 1998, and can be taken once a day. Extended-release Effexor is the first antidepressant to be approved for treatment of generalized anxiety disorder, although other antidepressants have also been authorized and are effective. Effexor XR is started at 37.5 mg, and raised 75 mg per week until 150 mg per day is reached. After that, if necessary, the dose is raised by 75 mg per day to a maximum of 375 mg per day.

Hypertension

As Wellbutrin's reputation has been tainted by the risk of seizures, so has Effexor's been by a connection with hypertension. In both cases, the hype is worse than the reality, but it is enough to dampen enthusiasm about each. Effexor has been shown to raise blood pressure primarily at doses over 225 mg a day. The increase is small and dose related. For example, if your blood pressure were 120/80 and you were taking 375 mg per day of Effexor, your blood pressure would increase by only 8 points.

In clinical trials, patients who are not medically healthy are typically excluded, and so the effect of Effexor on people with high blood pressure was not studied. Once hypertension occurs, the patient can be treated with an antihypertension drug, have the Effexor dose reduced, or change to another antidepressant. Hypertension, when it occurs, does so within two months of a given dose of Effexor having been established, and it is during this two-month period that patients require closest observation. People taking more than 225 mg a day of Effexor must take their blood pressure or have it taken, regularly. With many other new antidepressants and more than a dozen old ones, it is easy to see why Effexor is often not the first to be used.

Other Adverse Effects

Effexor is safe, even in overdose, from which people have survived thousands of milligrams without serious consequences. In fact, the nausea and vomiting that is induced by overdose serves to decrease the severity of the consequences.

The nausea, nervousness, dizziness, and sleepiness caused by Effexor at its starting dose of 37.5 or 75 mg a day is quite similar to the side effects of SSRIs. The incidence of side effects increases as the dose is raised. At the maximum dosage of 375 mg a day, about 40 percent of people taking the drug are nauseous, 13 percent sweating, 20 percent sleepy, 20 percent have dry mouth, 20 percent dizzy, 17 percent have headaches, and 10 percent suffer tremors. At lower doses, these unpleasant reactions are much less common. The abnormal ejaculation/orgasm, impotence, and lowered sexual desire caused by Effexor are the same as that for the SSRIs.

Stopping Effexor may cause more serious withdrawal reactions than from other antidepressants, starting in as few as eight hours. These include headaches, dizziness, depression, anxiety, numbness, and severe nausea. Sometimes 8 to 12 mg of Ondansetron (Zofran), an anti-nausea drug, is helpful. To avoid these withdrawal reactions, a very gradual decrease of the dose, perhaps 18.75 mg every five days, for as long as six weeks, may be required. The extended-release (XR) form of Effexor, while causing fewer side effects when started, produced the same number of withdrawal reactions.

Drug/Drug Interactions

Just as with the SSRIs, Effexor should not be taken with an MAOI. It should not be started for fourteen days after use of an MAOI is stopped, but, because of its short stay in the body, an MAOI can be taken seven days after use of Effexor is discontinued. Effexor does not seem to raise the blood levels of psychoactive drugs like the tricyclic desipramine, antipsychotics, and Tegretol. Tagamet taken together with Effexor raises Effexor's blood levels, which may mean that lower doses of Effexor will have to be used. No known interaction occurs between Effexor and lithium, alcohol, or benzodiazepines. Caution should be used when combining Effexor with other drugs, and as with all medications, be sure to consult your physician before doing so. An advantage of Effexor, like Celexa and Lexapro, is that it produces few drug/drug interactions.

Summary

Effexor seems a safe and effective antidepressant. The assertion that it is better than Prozac, because it affects two neurotransmitters (serotonin and norepinephrine), rather than one, remains unproven. Claims that it acts in a matter of days instead of weeks to combat depression may be an artifact of pushing high doses in time-limited trials with too little regard for the greater number of side effects thus caused. Proof for the notion that it is more effective in severely depressed patients also requires more than a study or two. And finally, the uncontrolled trial indicating that one third of previously untreatable depressives were helped by Effexor needs placebo-controlled replications, because new drugs usually help people due to the enthusiasm of both doctors and patients. If Effexor is truly more effective, especially in those who have not previously been helped by other treatments, then the fact that it must be taken more than once a day, except for the XR form, that its dose must be slowly raised, and that blood pressure must be carefully monitored, is a small price to pay for relief from pain and suffering caused by depression. Effexor has captured 13 percent of the antidepressant drug market, and is usually given only after another antidepressant has failed. It seems to alleviate chronic pain conditions, perhaps because of its dual serotonin-norepinephrine action.

Serzone (Nefazodone)

Serzone was released in 1995. It is similar in structure to Desyrel (trazodone), a drug that has many negative side effects, including drowsiness and faintness.

Having been withdrawn from the market in Europe and Canada, Serzone's days in America may be numbered. The *PDR* in 2002 added a long warning set off in heavy type and outlined in a box regarding "life-threatening hepatic failure" from Serzone, which occurs between two weeks and six months of the onset of treatment. The rate is very low ("1 case of liver failure resulting in death or transplant per 250,000 to 300,000 patient-years of Serzone treatment"), but is three to four times the normal rate of liver failure, and could be even higher due to underreporting. Patients must be alert for yellowing of the skin or whites of the eyes (jaundice), unusually dark urine, loss of appetite for several days or longer, nausea, and stomach pain. These signs must be reported immediately to physicians for blood tests measuring liver function (aspartate transaminase and alanine transaminase). Routine, periodic liver testing may not be as helpful in detecting this rare occurrence as being alert to newly arising clinical symptoms of liver disease. Of the 11 million people who have taken Serzone worldwide, there have been twenty-eight reported liver failures, and of these, eighteen have died.

Serzone, like the SSRIs, prevents serotonin reuptake, but it has a broader action in that it also blocks the part of the serotonin receptor responsible for insomnia, anxiety, and sexual dysfunction caused by the standard SSRIs, while activating only the clinically useful part of the receptor.

As Elliot S. Valenstein, a professor emeritus of psychology and neuroscience at the University of Michigan, has pointed out in his excellent book *Blaming the Brain,* "there is no convincing evidence that depressed people have a serotonin or norepinephrine deficiency." Why, then, are serotonin elevators effective as antidepressants? It must be that they start a chain of brain events we do not fully understand.

I regard the serotonin synapse the same way I think of my radio when it does not work—I hit it and it often starts broadcasting again. I have begun to believe that is what these antidepressants do to the synapse—they hit it. Thus, even the serotonin-lowering drug Tianeptine can be used in France as an antidepressant.

Serzone's Effectiveness

Serzone's effectiveness is equal to that of the tricyclic Tofranil and the SSRIs. The higher the dose of Serzone taken, the stronger its antidepressant power—up to 500 mg a day. At 600 mg a day, however, its effectiveness is weakened to that of a placebo. Since only nonresponders (those who don't get better on the drug) got the 600-mg dose in the studies, this finding may have little meaning beyond the fact that those who do not improve on 500 mg probably will not do so on 600 mg either, and so there is no advantage in raising the dose above 500 mg.

Within one week of starting Serzone, patients will notice an improvement in sleep and anxiety symptoms. The complete antidepressant response is no faster than that with other drugs. The value of Serzone in severe hospitalized patients requires further research. Continued treatment with Serzone produces protection against relapse comparable to that with other antidepressants.

Dosage

Serzone is started at 50 mg a day, and gradually increased to 150 mg one week later. The dose is then raised 50 to 75 mg per week, up to 300 mg per day. The dose is then gradually raised to a maximum of 500 mg a day. A greater response is expected at higher doses for those who do not improve initially. It is supplied in 50-, 100-, 150-, 200-, and 250-mg tablets.

Several researchers are experimenting giving 50 mg of Serzone at bedtime and gradually increasing the single dose every four days to achieve the same amount as that taken in divided portions twice daily. They believe it to be equally effective and without greater side effects. This has not yet become standard practice.

Side Effects

Serzone has no ill effect on the heart, even in overdosage. Dizziness, drowsiness, weakness, and lack of energy are its most common side effects, and occur more often than with any of the other new drugs, except perhaps Remeron. In one study A. Feiger et al. found Serzone to cause dizziness in 32 percent versus 7 percent on Zoloft. The reason for this is believed to be that it is the only one of the new drugs that blocks one of the serotonin receptors (serotonin-2) as well as the serotonin uptake pump. People are given the choice of being dizzy and sleepy or sexless, depending on whether they take Serzone or an SSRI.

Fortunately, the modifications to its parent, Desyrel (trazodone), have eliminated much of the drowsy, drugged feeling caused by the older compound. Desyrel also caused priapism (a permanent erection) in one of six thousand males treated. So far this has not yet been reported with Serzone.

The clear advantage of Serzone over the SSRIs, Wellbutrin, and Effexor is that it causes less sweating, anxiety, and sleeplessness. In fact, not only does the drug excel in these respects, it is better than a placebo, which means that it effectively combats anxiety in those who are depressed. Since a large number of depressed people are also anxious, this offers a distinct advantage. Also, since many require the help of a sleeping pill for several weeks until the nonsedating SSRI, Wellbutrin, or Effexor exerts its antidepressant action, Serzone's action as a sleep aid may be another advantage. Serzone has been shown in several studies to be associated with better sleep quality than Prozac.

Serzone and Sex

So far, it looks like Serzone has a low incidence of sexual side effects. One reason to withhold complete confidence in this assertion is that most studies are conducted for six weeks, and sexual side effects may occur after that initial six-week period. In addition, those who are seriously depressed do not care about sex or anything else, and may not report sexual dysfunction until they have recovered and become interested in sex again, and then find they cannot perform. There is also a difference between the ways in which men and women report sexual side effects. When a drug interferes with their sexual functioning, men are likely to report this side effect without being asked. Males complain spontaneously when they cannot get an erection or have difficulty ejaculating. Women, on the other hand, often attribute their loss of sexual interest or performance not to the drug but rather to being overworked or irritated with their husband or lover. Thus, they tend not to spontaneously report sexual side effects, and if the researchers do not specifically ask, they will underreport these side effects.

Wellbutrin is a drug to which you can change if the SSRIs have harmed your sexual functioning. Desyrel, the parent of Serzone, was found not to harm, and perhaps even to encourage, the sexual drive of women. In some cases, it went too far with men, producing permanent erection (priapism). So far it seems that Serzone is fulfilling its early promise as an effective antidepressant which harms sexual functioning about half as much as the SSRIs, but more than Wellbutrin.

Drug/Drug Interactions

The warning not to combine certain drugs with MAOIs extends to Serzone, although there is less potential danger than with the other antidepressants. Caution should be used when combining this drug with the antihistamines Seldane and Hismanal because of the unlikely but possible danger of increasing their blood levels, thus interfering with heart rhythm, which potentially can lead to ventricular tachycardia and death. Seldane and Hismanal have been withdrawn from the market. The combination of these drugs with the antifungal agent Nizoral (ketoconazole) or others and with the gastrointestinal agent Propulsid (cisapride) could also be toxic to the heart. The levels of Xanax and Halcion are raised four times by combining these drugs with Serzone. Serzone does not affect the asthma drug theophylline (Asbron) or the anticoagulant warfarin (Coumadin) or the anticonvulsant phenytoin (Dilantin), but can elevate levels of Tegretol. It does not increase the effects of alcohol and sedatives.

Summary

The advantages of Serzone are that it is sedating and therefore may calm anxiety and relieve insomnia more rapidly than other antidepressants. If excessive sweating is a problem, as it can be with many antidepressants, Serzone provides a good alternative. It makes more people dizzy than any of the other new antidepressants. It is usually taken twice daily, and the dosage gradually elevated to a peak of 500 mg. Recently it has been found that once-daily dosage is well tolerated and equally effective. Serzone can be initiated once daily and increased gradually or corrected from twice a day to a single nightly dosage. This need for gradual adjustment makes it more cumbersome to use than those SSRIs which require only one tablet a day. This combination has helped keep the drug's market share down at 4 percent. The black-box warning regarding severe liver toxicity, albeit rare, will most likely drive the market share further down.

Remeron (Mirtazapine)

Remeron, released in 1996, is unrelated to the SSRIs or other antidepressants. It enhances the amount of both serotonin and norepinephrine released into the synapse, but also blocks some of the target receptors of serotonin, which may account for why it, like Serzone, does not cause as much insomnia, anxiety, and sexual disturbance as the SSRIs. In addition, it affects several other neurotransmitters, which cause weight gain and mild sleepiness.

Remeron's Effectiveness

Five studies have shown Remeron's effectiveness in depressed patients equal to that of the tricyclic Elavil and superior to placebo, in the standard six-week controlled trials required by the FDA. As with the other new antidepressants, especially at the time of FDA approval, the main evidence of effectiveness has been obtained in outpatients. The smaller number of inpatient (and, most likely, more seriously ill) depressives studied shows Remeron equal to other antidepressants, but more research is necessary. Antidepressant and antianxiety effects can be seen as early as the second week.

Dosage

The recommended starting dose is one 15-mg tablet at bedtime, which if ineffective after two to four weeks can be raised gradually to 45 mg or more. The relationship between dosage and antidepressant response has not yet been established. Nonetheless, Remeron has the advantage of once-a-day dosage. The drug is available in 15- and 30-mg scored tablets, and 45-mg unscored tablets. It also comes in a rapid-dissolving wafer (Remeron SolTabs).

Side Effects

Remeron makes more than half of those who take it sleepy, especially in the first week of treatment, thus the recommendation that it be taken at bedtime. Going to work the next morning or being alert is not a problem because its sedative effect is not very strong. Nonetheless, care should be taken when driving. Sleepiness from antidepressants relieves insomnia at night and is usually gone the next day, especially after several weeks. Remeron causes about 10 percent to feel weakness and lack of energy. Appetite increase was reported in 17 percent and weight gain in 12 percent of patients in the brief six-week controlled studies, but in the months and years of normal clinical usage about 20 percent gain weight. Dry mouth is a common (25 percent) early side effect of Remeron, but it is usually mild and subsides in a few weeks. Nausea, vomiting, tremor, increased sweating, and insomnia are much less compared to the SSRIs, while weight gain, daytime sleepiness, and flulike symptoms are higher with Remeron.

Remeron and Sex

In the premarketing assessment of 2,796 patients, abnormal ejaculation was found to be rare (fewer than 1 in 1,000 patients), impotence infrequent (1 in 100 to 1 in 1,000 patients) and no mention is made of loss of sexual drive or orgasm potential. While the sexual side effects are less than those caused by the SSRIs, it is almost certain there will be more than reported in the six-week prerelease studies. Remeron has reversed SSRI-caused sexual side effects.

Other Adverse Effects

Severe Decrease in White Blood Cell Count

Three patients (1.1 per thousand) developed white counts below 500 (normal 3,800) during prerelease clinical trials. This occurrence is rare, but if you get a sore throat, fever, or other sign of infection, your doctor should test your blood. If the count is low, Remeron must be discontinued. While most antidepressant drugs lower the white count on rare occasions, none warn of its most severe form, agranulocytosis (a count below 500), in bold type in the *PDR*. Since 1996, when the drug was released, the initial concerns about low white blood cell counts with resulting dangerous infections and possible fatalities have not been substantiated, and the drug seems safe.

MAO Inhibitors

As with all the other new antidepressants, the manufacturer recommends Remeron not be used in combination with an MAOI.

Cholesterol Increases

Fifteen percent of patients treated with Remeron had up to a 20 percent increase of their nonfasting cholesterol level. This is twice the incidence seen on placebo and Elavil. I do not know how much of a problem this will prove to be, but it is something to be alert about when taking the drug for a long time.

Discontinuation of Treatment

Patients having to discontinue treatment within six weeks because of adverse effects number the same 16 percent occurring with other new antidepressants, and no doubt the number would have risen if observations had continued for a whole year, perhaps to the 30 to 35 percent level seen with others of these drugs. Remeron causes sleepiness, weight gain, dizziness, dry mouth, constipation, feelings of weakness, and debility, which lead to discontinuation in six weeks, and perhaps unknown late-occurring side effects, which would cause more patients to stop.

Drug/Drug Interactions

Remeron, because of its sedative side effects, probably will not mix very well with alcohol or Valium. Like all new antidepressants, it should not be taken with MAOIs. It can be combined safely with other psychiatric drugs, and is easy to do so with other antidepressants.

Overdose

Experience with Remeron is sparse in this area. The one death in twelve during the prerelease clinical trials occurred in a patient who also ingested Elavil. The eleven who took only Remeron recovered uneventfully. Overdose causes drowsiness, memory impairment, disorientation, rapid pulse, but so far there are no reports of serious effects on the heart or brain.

Summary

The search for more effective and better tolerated antidepressants goes on. The SSRIs cause more gastrointestinal upset, agitation, insomnia, and sexual disturbance than does

Remeron. Remeron is the first (perhaps the last) member of a new class of drugs, the noradrenaline (norepinephrine) and serotonin specific (*not* reuptake inhibitor) antidepressants (NaSSAs). Remeron acts by increasing norepinephrine and serotonin release, while partially blocking the side-effect aspect but not the therapeutic aspect of serotonin. It is no more effective than the SSRIs, but causes fewer sexual side effects, while substituting the danger of weight gain, mild dry mouth, and drowsiness.

Cymbalta (Duloxetine)

I am about to tell you all I have read about a soon-to-be-released norepinephrine-serotonin-balanced potential blockbuster of a drug with a predicted market value of $3 billion, Eli Lilly's replacement for the amount lost when Prozac became generic. But I must confess up front that I have never prescribed this potential powerhouse to a single patient. Let me tell you why.

I am a clinician who sees real patients in a book-lined, old-fashioned office, my sole source of income. I have been involved in teaching and writing about psychiatric drugs since my first article was published in the prestigious American Medical Association's *Archives of General Psychiatry* in 1963 entitled "Massive Doses of Chlorpromazine." This journal is refereed, which means an article must be approved before publication by expert reviewers chosen without the author's knowledge. But I have decided not to take money from drug companies, and thus cannot participate in the prerelease trials of Cymbalta, for which I would be well paid. I have the Harvard Medical School credentials and the experience and bibliography necessary to be involved, but have elected to remain separate from the early testing. Why not close this book and find one by an expert who has? Here is why you should not.

The old cliché has it that "he who has the gold makes the rules." The prerelease trial is paid for and managed by the drug company. I am sorry to say that some of the written reports sponsored by Lilly are filled with speculations that have little or no scientific support. First let me describe the process, and then I will tell you what has been disappointing.

Lilly's methods are no different from those of other pharmaceutical companies launching a new drug, or in this case, an antidepressant. About a dozen leading depression researchers are recruited to a Cymbalta advisory board to help assess the drug. They are paid a fee, receive traveling expenses, and most important, receive support for their research, which sustains their academic medical careers, which give them their professional status. This can get a bit out of hand, as reported by the *Boston Globe* in 1999 regarding Dr. Martin Keller, a Brown University professor and chairman of their psychiatric department, who earned $842,000 that year, $556,000 of which came from consulting for drug companies. I doubt that his story is uniquely different from the other members of a drug advisory board, a group of what I suspect to be twelve millionaires. There have been debates among ethicists regarding whether pharmaceutical support influences the direction of allegedly pure psychiatric research, but this subject is out of my clinician's area of expertise, and I leave such ponderings to others.

Then the drug companies identify about two hundred top psychiatric thought leaders who are paid to put about twenty patients each on the new drug to try to work out dosage and record results both positive and negative. If my math is right, this amounts to 4,000 patients. Next, $500 each is paid to 600 doctors who agree to test five patients each, which should add another 3,000 patients. Finally, a large number of the biggest prescribers of antidepressants are approached with a chance to get ahead of all the other psychiatrists. By the day Cymbalta is officially launched, about 15,000 patients will have gotten it. Because I have chosen to remain outside of this prerelease juggernaut, I cannot prescribe the drug until the FDA officially puts it in drugstores.

There is an advantage to being on the sideline, besides

freedom from economic taint. It gives me a chance to closely read what the insiders write, to talk to them, several of whom I know personally, and to observe Lilly's premarketing advertising strategy. The FDA rules do not allow Lilly to market Cymbalta before it is officially approved for efficacy and safety. Furthermore, the FDA advisory committee negotiates with the company about what it will and will not be allowed to say in its advertising.

Lilly's prerelease "advertising" and strategy have been extremely interesting. It is subtle enough that it took me some time to put it together, but I think I have cracked the code. It's all out in published material. I have not relied on any leaks.

In 2000, the American Psychiatric Association's *DSM* IV Text Revision was published. This keeps with the pattern: *DSM* III, *DSM* III R (revised), *DSM* IV, *DSM* IV TR. The *DSM* IV TR contains a very interesting alteration in the list of symptoms of major depressive disorder, which now includes ". . . excessive worry over physical health, and complaints of pain (e.g., headaches or joint, abdominal or other pains)." I could see how this prepares the way for "a medication that treats all aspects of Major Depressive Disorder," including what has been newly added, making it more useful than its predecessors. Furthermore, Cymbalta balances its effects on norepinephrine and serotonin better than its predecessor, Effexor. The quotes are from Michael J. Detke, M.D., Ph.D., and others, writing on duloxetine (Cymbalta) in the April 2002 *Journal of Clinical Psychiatry*.

The trail continues in a curious ad that has been appearing for several months in a variety of psychiatric publications. The one I happen to be looking at right now is in the prestigious *American Journal of Psychiatry*, dated September 2003. In large type, the following appears: "Depression has long been defined by emotional symptoms, such as crying, loss of interest, worrying, and nervousness. But at Lilly, we're exploring the role not only of emotional symptoms, but also of physical symptoms in depression, such as vague aches and pains.

Depression is both emotional and physical. Patients may suffer the more painful physical symptoms in silence, unaware of their connection to depression. Nineteen million adults in the United States still suffer from a depressive disorder. Imbalance of Serotonin (5-HT) and norepinephrine (NE) may contribute to both the emotional and physical symptoms of depression. Depression hurts both emotionally and physically."

Why is Lilly spending all this money in one of psychiatry's most prestigious journals (I wonder what fee the journal collects for this ad)? It is to promote the "new" illness, *depression with physical complaints* (and perhaps without depressed mood), preparing the way for what they cannot yet say, and be in compliance with FDA rules: "prescribe Cymbalta." The letter of the law is being followed, if not the spirit.

From my seat on the sidelines, I begin to see what is happening. The target of this campaign is the overworked primary care physician who prescribes more antidepressants than all the expert psychiatrists and psychopharmacologists combined. These "gatekeepers" have too many patients and no time for each one. Those who come to them have been found not to present, the way psychiatric patients do, with mood symptoms such as loss of pleasure and interest, but with physical aches and pains for which frequently no medical cause can be found. They will certainly welcome Cymbalta, which purports to correct the alleged dysfunction in the pain pathways connecting the brain to the body. Once Cymbalta bolsters the ascending and descending nerve conduction routes of serotonin and norepinephrine, the person will begin to focus on the external world and stop being preoccupied with the frantic bodily messages arising from their allegedly imbalanced nerves, which are causing them headaches, stomachaches, and backaches. Cymbalta will encourage not only medical doctors, in general, but even psychiatric specialists to no longer foolishly view depression and painful physical symptoms as separate, but to be treated as one, and thus, cured. The *DSM* IV TR in 2000 has prepared the way. The marketers never seem to identify which physicians have been so stupid as not to notice that their patients with chronic pain might be depressed. In fact, even the much maligned primary care physician, who is often depicted in snotty psychiatric journals as not observing much of anything, has been giving Elavil (amtriptyline) to such patients for over forty years.

What, then, is Lilly up to? Without turning this into a Sherlock Holmes mystery novel, I suspect they aim to replace Elavil, as well as the benzodiazepines, with Cymbalta. Elavil is generic and it is a tricyclic, producing dry mouth, constipation, rapid heartbeat, and danger in overdose. This rarely if ever happens in the medical clinic to chronic pain patients on small 25- or 50-mg-per-day doses for years, but the aim is to substitute Cymbalta for this old drug.

Of course, it, too, has side effects, but more of this later. But I suspect even more of a target are the benzodiazepines, the Valium, Xanax, Klonopin, and Ativan, drugs that remain the largest prescribed group by medical doctors. I must confess I am a little cynical. It is hard to be against progress and hope. No one honors the prophet who says the Dow Jones average will go down 500 points or more, and then is proven right. I do not wish to be an old grump about Cymbalta. Since after ten new antidepressants, Lilly says in its ad that 19 million Americans remain depressed, and since the drugs have a 65 percent response rate, and a lot lower cure rate, it is hard to see how Cymbalta will be penicillin. People who have had pain with or without depression for years do not suddenly get cured. Rather, they are managed, hopefully, by family doctors with a little kindness and concern for them, and not excessively driven by the MBA's passion for time and efficiency, or Dr. Michael Detke's science-lite regarding pain pathways being balanced by the most balanced of new antidepressants, Cymbalta.

Nonetheless, this will be a blockbuster drug. Lilly knows its audience. Patients will demand it because of direct TV and print advertising. Doctors will want to try the latest. Elavil is generic and has no Lilly to champion it. The benzodiazepines have been dunned as addictive, although they are only so in addicts. No thirty-year-old, well-dressed, good-looking blonde sales representatives will give physicians pens, coffee mugs, expensive dinners, tickets to the ballgame, or journal articles providing them with the latest information. The continuing medical education (CME) credits required to be assembled to renew their medical licenses every two years will not feature lectures on the benzodiazepines or Elavil or amtriptyline, but on Cymbalta. The academic-industrial complex will not be denied.

Efficacy

The standard of two controlled studies proving Cymbalta superior to placebo in the treatment of depression has been met and exceeded, and release of the drug is imminent. (There are four of them.) The fact that the drug failed to beat placebo on two other similar studies goes unmentioned. A one-year uncontrolled investigation finds it safe in the longer term. Over three thousand people have already taken Cymbalta. Prerelease studies are not required to compare the effectiveness of a new antidepressant to those already available. The half-life of Cymbalta is twelve hours, which initially frightened the company with the specter of twice-a-day dosage. Fortunately, Dr. Detke and his group have come to the rescue and found it equally effective when given in 60-mg doses once a day. Presumably, they say, it hangs around in the brain longer than it does in the bloodstream.

The effect on serotonin and norepinephrine begins immediately, unlike Effexor, which at lower doses is an SSRI, and affects norepinephrine only at higher doses. Cymbalta allegedly does not cause hypertension, unlike Effexor, in which it occurs in 13 percent at higher doses. Cymbalta has no cardiovascular effects and does not disturb cardiac conduction, as the tricyclic antidepressant Elavil does. The dropout rate because of side effects was comparable to the SSRIs, at around 14 percent. The most frequent side effects were mild to moderate nausea (13 to 25 percent), which usually subsides in a week.

The prerelease scientific evidence of efficacy stops with eight-week double-blind trials, but this does not stop the speculations about how this drug *may* compare to the existing ten. Because of its more balanced "dual" (norepinephrine-serotonin) action, it may be more rapidly effective. The five-day to three-week or longer lag time between the start of medication and significant clinical result is a big problem with all antidepressants. It also is alleged to cause more remissions (read cures) than its predecessors. Remember, this is more speculation. On what is it based? It is based on "estimated probabilities of remission," as calculated from the eight-week studies by statisticians. No one asked a patient whether they were cured of their depression. This was all calculated mathematically, derived from our old friend, the Hamilton Depression Rating scale. If Max Hamilton were still alive, I suspect he would sneer at this claim of cure.

Chronic Pain

It is hard to shock me, but here is what backs up the claim that Cymbalta has a unique advantage in the treatment of chronic pain. It is the eight-week Hamilton Depression Rating scale's item 13. Item 13 inquires about physical symptoms, including backaches, headaches, and muscle aches. Dr. Detke and his group are particularly impressed, they write, by the striking effect on pain "given that the population was NOT selected for pain . . ." Not a single patient was interviewed and asked about whether or not they suffered years of backaches, headaches, and stomachaches. Nowhere is it stated that they were the people chronically depressed and physically distressed without demonstrable cause that plague internists and make their patients suffer. In fact, chronic depressives are excluded from all prerelease studies because of the need to assemble a pure sample for study. The HAM-D-17 was broken down by Dr. Detke and his associates into five subscales plus item 13 (listed separately), and the patients improved on all six of them. The improvement on three others of the six items appears much more striking than that on item 13, which was, in fact, the weakest. This is marketing, not science, and Lilly will nonetheless have its blockbuster because it has captured the psychiatric thought leaders, and sent out the army of good-looking representatives, and funded the medical school lunches and CME courses. Only the journal's front-page conclusion will be read by a small percentage of physicians who see it at all, and it states the following, which I quote in its entirety, "Duloxetine (Cymbalta), 60 mg/day, is a well-tolerated and effective treatment for MDD that reduces painful symptoms. These findings suggest that duloxetine may be a first-line treatment for MDD and associated painful physical symptoms" (*Journal of Clinical Psychiatry* 2002; 63: 308–315).

Adverse Events

Only insomnia, weakness, and fatigue occur more often with Cymbalta than with placebo. The drug is safe for the EKG and the cardiovascular system overall. Mild to moderate nausea occurs in about 25 percent, and is transient. No hypertension was observed from its norepinephrine effect.

Summary

The promise of more rapid treatment response and higher remission (i.e., cure) rate (as defined by a HAM-D-17 score under 7 within eight weeks, rather than by direct questioning of actual clinic or office patients over months and years) has been heard before when a new drug was launched. "Remission" is a tricky word, which I plan to look into further in the section on Treatment-Resistant Depression. Since there has never been an agreed-to psychiatric definition of "normal," it is hard to judge what a cure is when there is no thermometer by which to measure it. The pain story is unsupported by real clinical or scientific data. Not a single patient has told any interviewer that their back pain is gone, their headache subsided, their stomach is feeling better.

Event	Cymbalta	Placebo	Tricyclic Antidepressant	Prozac
Dry mouth	27%	61 (15%)	174 (35%)	15 (6.9%)
Constipation	11.4%	36 (9%)	94 (19%)	12 (5.6%)
Nausea	25%	27 (7%)	45 (9%)	40 (18.5%)
Insomnia	20%	28 (7%)	42 (8%)	23 (10.6%)
Dizziness	15.7%	23 (6%)	64 (13%)	13 (6%)
Tremor	11	(3%)	43 (9%)	15 (7%)
Sleepiness	18.6%	29 (7%)	38 (8%)	10 (5%)
Headache	20%	56 (14%)	62 (12%)	43 (20%)
Sweating	18.6%	31 (8%)	84 (17%)	15 (7%)
Rapid pulse	2%	10 (2.5%)	40 (8%)	4 (2%)
Low blood pressure	0%	9 (2%)	25 (5%)	1 (0.5%)
High blood pressure	0%	2 (0.5%)	8 (1.6%)	2 (1%)
Urination impaired		6 (1.5%)	14 (3%)	1 (0.5%)
Impotence		0	1 (0.2%)	2 (0.9%)
Sexual function abnormal		2 (0.5%)	3 (0.6%)	2 (0.9%)

Summary of Wellbutrin, Effexor, Serzone, Remeron, and Cymbalta

The following table compares some of the main characteristics of Wellbutrin, Effexor, Serzone, Remeron, and Cymbalta.

	Wellbutrin	Effexor	Serzone	Remeron	Cymbalta
Mechanism of action	Unknown* Weak dopamine and norepinephrine reuptaker inhibitor	Norepinephrine and serotonin reuptake inhibitor	Two actions on serotonin and norepinephrine reuptake inhibitor	Increases release of norepinephrine and serotonin	Norepinephrine and serotonin reuptake inhibitor
Dosage frequency	3 ×/day 1 × day XL	2–3 ×/day 1 × day XR	2–3 ×/day	1 ×/day	1 ×/day
Total amount daily	225–450 mg	75–375 mg	200–500 mg	15–45 mg	60–120 mg
Possible side effects					
Sexual dysfunction	No	Yes	Less	Less	Yes
Dizziness, sleepiness	No	Yes	Yes	Yes	Yes
Anxiety, agitation, insomnia	Yes	Yes	No	No	Yes
Seizures	Yes	No	No	No	No
Hypertension	Infrequent	Yes	No	No	No
Weight gain	Infrequent	Infrequent	Infrequent	Yes	Unknown

*The metabolism of Wellbutrin is not fully understood

Clinicians have been trained to listen to patients, not statisticians. I hope they do not succumb to the siren lure of what is supposed to be science, and forget their primary skill, for which they have been carefully schooled. I hope Cymbalta gives the long suffering complete pain relief. If it does, neither the patient nor the doctor will need randomly controlled, double-blind studies to confirm it. None was ever necessary for morphine. Both doctor and patient immediately knew that it was effective. The statistician is only required when the clinical effect is weaker. In the case of Cymbalta, I believe mathematics has been falsely represented as testifying to the drug's unique action. All eleven new antidepressants, in those studies in which they manage to be more effective than placebo, must be compared to one another regarding item 13 of the HAM-D-17. If Cymbalta ends up in first place by a wide margin, I will then be happily convinced of its unparalleled action. Or better still, if the back pain of many long-suffering patients goes away, I will be even more impressed.

The hope that biological probes will be developed to show which depressions are serotonergic or noradrenergic (norepinephrine) in origin remains a fallacy in my opinion based on the repeated unwillingness to face a fundamental fact. After almost fifty years no chemical deficiency in either of these neurotransmitters has been consistently shown to exist. That either a serotonin, norepinephrine, or dual antidepressant relieves depression does not prove the condition was caused by a lack of the neurotransmitter any more than when aspirin relieves a headache it provides evidence that the pain in the head was caused by a lack of aspirin. Regarding the mechanism of action of an antidepressant as evidence of the cause of the depression is silly. Yet the serotonin and norepinephrine believers persist in doing so. Some experts proclaim that serotonin is "associated primarily with mood and norepinephrine is most closely associated with energy and drive." In my opinion this assertion is very unlikely to prove true. I have heard similar ones for over forty years which, based on too little solid evidence, have ended up as nothing more than advertising copy and entries on long academic curriculum vitae. For one thing, it seems impossible to influence norepinephrine without affecting serotonin as well. The brain seems to balance the two such that when a drug changes one, the other is also altered.

We need a drug that so far does not exist and perhaps never will, one that provides a better quality of life for depressed people, too many of whom have partially recovered after taking the previous antidepressants so they are able to sleep, eat, and work while feeling less depressed, but nonetheless remain impaired with few friends and an empty social life. The two new antidepressants, Lexapro and Cymbalta, are as effective as the previous nine. Their long-term safety is still unknown.

The following conclusions can be drawn about these new drugs:

- They are all equally effective.
- More work will be required to prove the claim that Effexor is the most curative or that Cymbalta has a unique effect on pain.
- Studies show that Wellbutrin, perhaps Serzone, and possibly Remeron have the fewest sexual side effects.
- The danger of seizures from Wellbutrin can be minimized through careful dosing.
- Hypertension, sexual dysfunction, and anxiety/insomnia are drawbacks of Effexor.
- Dizziness or feelings of weakness and lack of energy are problems with Serzone and Remeron, but they do not raise blood pressure (as does Effexor) and do not make people feel agitated and "wired" (as do all of the others).
- Remeron has the advantage of once-a-day dosage, but weight gain from it may be a drawback.

Whether Cymbalta's dual action (serotonin and norepinephrine) make it more rapidly acting, more likely to cure rather than merely improve, and cause it to be uniquely effective for headaches, backaches, stomachaches, sleep disturbances, and fatigue, and thus a drug of choice for primary caregivers, remains to be proven. Currently, these assertions are based on statistical extrapolations from eight-week, double-blind, prerelease studies. If these mathematical fantasies become clinical realities, this drug will make a significant contribution. I worry that overworked primary care physicians, impatient with complaints for which no physical cause can be found, will listen to Lilly's sales representatives, respond to patient's demands for the latest, and thoughtlessly prescribe Cymbalta. I guess that might not be so bad if physicians didn't pompously write articles about "evidence-based medicine." As long as everybody understands that hope and enthusiasm do a lot to help, and stops pontificating about science, little harm will be done and probably a whole lot of good. When the excitement wears down after several years, there will still be 19 million or more depressed people in the United States awaiting the next drug.

The whole process would be a lot more humane if the doctors didn't throw a pill at those who suffer chronic pain and depression, and instead took the time to listen to their concerns and help them find a more constructive way to live their lives rather than trying to extract a little care, and perhaps substitute for love, by having symptoms in a busy physician's office.

Some of these drugs have advantages over the SSRIs regarding activation (anxiety, insomnia) or sexual dysfunction, all but Remeron and Effexor XR (extended release) have the disadvantages of multiple dosing and of requiring close monitoring for dose elevation to achieve maximum efficacy, and each has a drawback: Wellbutrin may cause seizures, Effexor may raise blood pressure, Serzone and Remeron may cause dizziness or feelings of weakness and loss of energy. But more important than these side effect differences (in some cases, minor), the main drawback of all these new antidepressants as well as the old ones is that about 30 percent of people do not respond, and another 30 percent do so only partially, and are not completely cured. It is for these people who continue suffering that more effective treatments must be found. Chapter 7 is devoted to the treatment-resistant depressed individual.

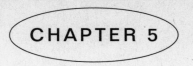

CHAPTER 5

The Benzodiazepines

Since these antianxiety agents have been available since the 1960s, I will confine my discussion to those of which you might have heard. They are Valium (diazepam), Ativan (lorazepam), Serax (oxazepam), Xanax (alprazolam), and Klonopin (clonazepam). All of them exist in generic form, except when a new method of administration is formulated, such as Xanax XR, which permits once-daily dosing, or Klonopin Wafer, which can be taken under the tongue. The table on the next page summarizes the strengths and dose range of each, the speed with which it acts, and how long the effect lasts.

Uses and Effectiveness

All five of the drugs listed are equally effective in the treatment of anxiety and as sleep aids. Since none cures anxiety or insomnia, a return of long-standing symptoms can be anticipated when the drug is discontinued. In studies of long-term benzodiazepine users, patients who received unknown placebo

Name Brand/Generic	Tablet/Capsule Availability	Dose Range	How Fast They Work	Duration of Action (hrs)	Comparison Dose (mg)
Valium (diazepam)	*Tablets:* 2, 5, 10 mg	4–40	Fast	30–60	5
Ativan (lorazepam)	*Tablets:* 0.5, 1, 2 mg *Oral Solution:* 2 mg/ml (30 mml)	1–6	Intermediate	10–20	1
Serax (oxazepam)	*Capsules:* 10, 15, 30 mg	15–120	Slow	8–12	15
Xanax (alprazolam)	*Tablets:* 0.25, 0.5, 1, 2 mg *Oral Solution:* 1 mg/ml (30 mml)	Anxiety 0.75–4	Intermediate	4–6	0.5
Xanax XR (alprazolam)	0.5, 1, 2, 3 mg	Panic dis. 1.5–10	Intermediate to slow	9–16	0.5
Klonopin (clonazepam)	0.5, 1, 2 mg	0.5–4	Intermediate	30–40	0.25
Klonopin Wafer	0.124, 0.25, 0.5, 1, 2 mg	0.5–4	Intermediate	30–40	0.125

substitution had symptoms recur, whereas those continued on active medication did not.

Anxiety

There are two types of anxiety. Situational anxiety, which is appropriate to the stressor being faced and stimulates coping behavior, such as practice, studying, or rehearsal, and pathological anxiety, which involves excessive worry for most of six months. The worry in generalized anxiety disorder (GAD) is associated with feeling on edge or restless, fatigue, difficulty concentrating, irritability, muscle tensions, or sleep disturbance. The pathological anxiety causes significant distress and interferes with social or work functioning. There are many ways to treat GAD, and one of these is through the use of the benzodiazepines. If this course is decided upon, it is often impossible to predict how long it will be needed. For some, months or years will be required, much as with insulin for diabetics. Medically ill patients are often appropriately prescribed benzodiazepines, which continue to be effective, for the anxious component of their conditions.

Depression

Reports of controlled studies of benzodiazepines in the treatment of depressive disorders are mixed. A main reason for this is the continuing vagueness of the term "depression," even into the modern era of *DSM* IV TR. Severe depression, with its many previous and current appellations ("endogenous," "autonomous," major affective disorder, psychotic, melancholia), responds better to antidepressant medications than it does to antianxiety agents. But, judging from the 25 million people now on antidepressants in the United States, I suspect only 10 to 20 percent are severe depressives. One indication of the laxity with which the term "depression" is used in the typical modern medical and psychiatric nonhospital practice is the growth in the number of people so diagnosed. Since 1950, the number of patients termed depressed has grown from the rare 50 to 100 per million to 100,000 per million, a thousandfold increase. The reason, in my opinion, is not that physicians have become more skillful in their diagnostic acumen, but that the ground rules have changed. Fifty years ago, patients considered depressed were immobilized in hospital beds, refusing food and actively suicidal. Today's "depressed" *out*patient is unhappy, dragging to work and at home, but nonetheless able to struggle through. While technically sharing the same list of *DSM* IV TR symptoms as those fifty years ago, the group is not only vastly increased in number, but also responds equally well to the benzodiazepines as to the antidepressants. The 1950 hospitalized depressive responded much better to the antidepressants and much less to the antianxiety agents. The benzodiazepines are particularly helpful in depressed patients who are also anxious, agitated, suffer insomnia, and whose response to the stress of medical illness causes them not only to suffer, but at times to make the medical condition worse, such as in hypertension or back pain.

Other Uses of the Benzodiazepines

In the mid-1970s, Valium was the most widely prescribed drug available in the United States. It was, and often still is, used in almost all psychiatric disorders, anxiety accompanying medical illness, compulsive disorders, muscle spasticity, involuntary movement disorders, and detoxification from alcohol and other substances. It has use in surgery, chemotherapy, and dentistry. The benzodiazepines continue to this day to be the most frequently prescribed psychoactive medications in America. In the early 1980s, Xanax was released, and by the end of the eighties had displaced Valium as the most commonly prescribed antianxiety agent.

Benzodiazepines in Panic Disorder

Xanax was recognized as effective in panic disorder, while Valium was not considered. The reason for this is that Valium was available almost twenty years before panic disorder was defined in 1980 by the *DSM* III. In a study reported by Russell Noyes, Jr., M.D., et al., in 1996 in the *Journal of Clinical Psychiatry* comparing the two, Valium proved every bit the equal of Xanax in the treatment of panic disorder. They said that long-term benzodiazepine use might lead to "dependency and withdrawal if . . . not tapered properly," and had adverse sedative side effects. What they did not say was what dependency means. Does it mean requiring long-term usage in a chronic condition? If so, then would SSRI treatment be quicker? They never said, and provided no evidence. If benzodiazepines upset people when suddenly withdrawn after months or years of use, is this not also true of SSRIs? If benzodiazepines have sedative side effects, don't SSRIs have them, too? Are the physicians and patients who prefer the "rapid onset of action of the benzodiazepines" to the newer SSRIs, "which can take weeks to provide any benefit" just being old-fashioned and resistant to expert practice guidelines? The rapid effect allows many people to take benzodiazepines on an as-needed basis. Panic disorder patients discontinued SSRIs 52 percent of the time due to "adverse side effects," the *American Journal* article noted, whereas only 7 percent of the benzodiazepine patients did so. The Harvard/Brown Anxiety Research Project, responsible for the *American Journal* report, recommended patient education regarding SSRI side effects and slowness of action. Perhaps it is the experts who need the education. Finally, the Harvard/Brown group admit there is "no large controlled comparison study [that] has been conducted to examine the superiority of SSRIs over benzodiazepines for the treatment of panic disorder." They want the gap between clinical research and actual delivery of care to be minimized. I would like to ask them to what clinical research they refer. Unfortunately, there is none.

Side Effects

Drowsiness and sleepiness are the most commonly reported side effects. These usually decrease with time and are minimized by starting with relatively low doses. In most people, a daily amount is achieved, which produces maximum clinical effect with minimal side effects. In those who feel tired, drowsy, have trouble remaining awake or concentrating, feel slowed down, or have trouble balancing, they will find these to subside, especially if the dose is temporarily lowered. A few who are sedated temporarily have trouble acquiring or remembering information. Some studies have shown an increased number of automobile accidents among benzodiazepine users. It is hard to know what to make of these findings, since it could as easily be the mental disorder for which the drug is being taken as much as the benzodiazepine itself that is responsible.

Tolerance, Abuse, Addiction, and Dependence

Tolerance

Tolerance is much more likely to the sedative side effects of these drugs than it is to the antianxiety effect, but the latter occasionally happens. Prozac "poop out" syndrome also occasionally occurs. In fact, all psychiatric drugs sometimes stop working. I know of no evidence that benzodiazepines are more likely to stop being effective than any of the others, or that they lead to tolerance, and invite escalation of dosage to re-create the original therapeutic effect.

Abuse

This term refers to the nontherapeutic taking of drugs for pleasure, deliberate intoxication, and to achieve a "high." The rare benzodiazepine abuser is usually someone who has also excessively drunk alcohol and taken a variety of illegal substances. Such individuals use very high doses and spend hours in search of legal and/or illegal drugs, which interferes with their work and relationships. No single benzodiazepine is more likely to risk abuse, although the rapid-onset ones are preferred by abusers.

For patients who are anxious and have no abuse history, appropriate benzodiazepine therapeutic use almost never leads to abuse or misuse.

There is a widespread belief among doctors that long-term use of benzodiazepines can be addicting. The fact is that only chronic substance abusers abuse them. Nonabusers using them for painful anxieties and chronic insomnias, even when continuing the medication for months and years, do not abuse them. Abuse means, as I said earlier, the nonthera-peutic taking of a drug for pleasure, to become intoxicated, and to get high. GAD patients do not escalate their benzodiazepine dose, get intoxicated, or become high from the drug, and do not spend their days seeking ever-larger quantities. Then why does the notion persist that benzodiazepines can be addicting? I believe it is due to the influence of addiction specialists, who see only alcoholics and narcotics addicts. They may also take huge doses of Valium or Xanax. The trouble is addiction specialists frighten many other doctors, sometimes triggering fantasies of being persecuted by the narcotics bureau. The average family doctor or psychiatrist need not worry, nor should the patient. No one will become addicted. The suffering person will just be helped.

Dependence and Withdrawal

Physical dependence on long-term, especially high-dose benzodiazepine use does occur, accompanied by a withdrawal syndrome of sweating, insomnia, gastrointestinal discomfort, rapid heartbeat, and hypersensitivity to light and sound. The withdrawal is mild, self-limited, without long-lasting effects, and is most likely to be more severe if the drug is abruptly stopped. Benzodiazepines are not unique in this regard. Any long-term, high-dose psychoactive drug should be gradually tapered. Cutting it cold turkey is unpleasant and sometimes dangerous. Psychological dependence implies that people like taking their benzodiazepines. It does not mean abuse or misuse. If a patient has been extremely worried for months, suffering panic attacks; has aches, pains, and muscle tension; has difficulty enjoying his family, friends; and is hampered at work, and if Valium or Xanax gives great relief, then of course that person will want to continue the drug.

Widespread Benzodiazepine Use Continues

After more than forty years, without benefit of TV or print advertising, and despite derision from experts and ominous warnings from addiction specialists, these drugs continue to be the number one psychoactives prescribed for a combination of bad and good reasons. The bad reasons are physician habit, laziness, and patients' habit (called dependence). The good reasons are their effectiveness, rapid onset of action, ability to be used on an as-needed basis, and their remarkable safety and lack of side effects.

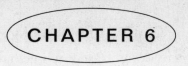

CHAPTER 6

The Treatment of Insomnia

About half of America experiences transient insomnia in times of acute stress, and 10 to 20 percent suffer from it chronically. Before any treatment can be considered, its cause must be carefully investigated. Insomnia is characterized by difficulty falling asleep or staying asleep, awakening too early, or being unable to go back to sleep if awakened. Some individuals say they get no rest at all, or feel unrefreshed afterward. Daytime functioning may be impaired as a result, accompanied by irritability, difficulty concentrating, headaches, grogginess, dozing off easily at one's desk or while driving, and fatigue. Social relationships and work capacity may be harmed, job performance deteriorate, and absenteeism increase.

People most likely to suffer insomnia are the elderly, females, shift workers, and those with medical and psychiatric disorders. It is often difficult to decide whether lack of sleep is the cause or the result of depression, anxiety, or alcohol abuse.

Causes of Insomnia

About 80 percent of depressed people have trouble falling asleep, have trouble staying asleep, or awaken too early. Anxious patients also have problems getting to sleep, and they experience disrupted sleep. In some, sleep panic attacks occur. Nightmares disturb the sleep of posttraumatic stress disorder sufferers.

Sleep is transiently disturbed by job loss, bereavement, or hospitalization. Many medical and psychiatric drugs disturb sleep, including antidepressants, diuretics, stimulants, and corticosteriods. Other intruders upon rest include restless legs syndrome, the snoring or breathing pauses of sleep apnea, circadian rhythm disturbances due to travel or shift work, chronic pain, heart and lung disease, hyperthyroidism, and the hot flashes of menopause. Drug and alcohol abuse also interfere with sleep. Insomnia, therefore, results from multiple causes which must be carefully evaluated before treatment is begun. Transient insomnia usually requires brief treatment, sometimes accompanied by medication, while what is secondary to pain or other causes is dealt with by resolving whatever is disrupting the individual's sleep. Primary insomnia, a diagnosis made in which sleep is disturbed for no apparent reason, can be made worse by too much coffee or alcohol, daytime napping, and by becoming anxious and preoccupied with the sleep problem itself. In those who become frightened and preoccupied with whether they will be able to fall asleep, their natural sleepiness is overcome by worry, which keeps them awake. Some people think they are not sleeping, but observation in a sleep lab reveals they are getting as much sleep as normal, but do not realize it. Some get the right amount of sleep at the wrong time, children and adolescents go to bed late and get up late, and the elderly are liable to fall asleep and wake up too early.

The Treatment of Chronic Primary Insomnia

I will focus here on the medication treatment of chronic primary insomnia, although good sleep practices, a regular bedtime, avoiding daytime naps, getting sufficient exercise (but not just before bedtime), limiting alcohol and caffeine, allowing time to wind down, and trying to worry less about the process are very important. The medications most commonly used are benzodiazepines or two nonbenzodiazepines (perhaps soon to be joined by several others), which act on part of the same receptor but are technically not benzodiazepines because of their chemical structure. The main differences among the drugs listed in the table are speed of absorption and duration of action. Those most rapidly absorbed can be taken at bedtime, while the others must be ingested an hour or two before. The long-acting ones assure a full night's sleep, but may cause morning hangover; the ultrashort-acting ones may be taken in the middle of the night if the person is unable to fall asleep without medication or wakes up and is unable to fall back asleep, but when ingested early may lead to awakening in the middle of the night. The two new drugs being developed and awaiting release to join Ambien and Sonata are Estorra and Indiplon.

The special binding to a part of the benzodiazepine receptor by Ambien and Sonata, instead of to all of it as traditional benzodiazepines do, is called a breakthrough by some, and is said to produce fewer side effects because of more selective modulation of gamma-aminobutyric acid (GABA) receptors in the brain. Other experts find this special binding to be of no clinical value.

Prescribing Hypnotics

All of the drugs described are benzodiazepines or slight modifications of them. Most commonly used for the brief treatment of insomnia, they are typically given periodically for subsequent brief periods. Some chronic insomniacs require

Hypnotic Agents

Generic	Trade	Onset	Duration of Action (hrs)	Strength Available (mg)	Dose Range (mg)
Benzodiazepines					
Flurazepam	Dalamane	Rapid	48	15, 30	15–30
Temazepam	Restoril	Intermediate	8–12	7.5, 15	7.5–30
Triazolam	Halcion	Rapid	6	0.125, 0.25, 0.5	0.125–0.5
Benzodiazepine-like					
Zolpidem	Ambien	Rapid	2.5	5, 10	5–10
Zaleplon	Sonata	Rapid	1	5, 10, 20	5–10, occasionally 20

months or years of continuous benzodiazepine treatment, which continues to be effective and is not accompanied by abusive escalation and addiction. There is some debate about whether long-term hypnotics ought to be prescribed to the minority who are known to abuse drugs or alcohol. Some authorities say never, and others say carefully. All of the benzodiazepines listed in the previous chapter can also be used in the treatment of insomnia.

The conscientious physician explores all causes of insomnia before making the diagnosis of chronic primary insomnia, and then employs all behavioral methods available to help chronic insomniacs sleep medication free. But despite these efforts, about 10 to 20 percent continue to suffer severe, chronic lack of sleep. The physician is then faced with the difficult choice between medicating the individual for months or years, or allowing the chronic insomniac to live untreated with the consequences of sleeplessness. These are, as I have discussed, far reaching and include depression, daytime dozing, automobile accidents, irritable effects on work colleagues and family, inferior performance leading to job loss, narrowing of social life, chronic alcoholism or drug abuse, and problems with spouses and children. A chronically tired person with dark rings under his eyes and a headache gets few promotions at work, and is a strain to the family.

If the decision to medicate is forced upon the physician when other means have failed, then the popular bias against the benzodiazepines must be overcome in the minds of the physician and the patient. For those who have been on benzodiazepines for years, an attempt at gradual tapering off to see if the drug is still necessary can be tried. But if this fails, and it often does, because of persistent insomnia, chronic severe anxiety, panic disorder, or depression, then a benzodiazepine or benzodiazepine-like medication ought not be regarded as evidence of physiologic dependence, but as required because of the continued severity of symptoms. If the patient is still suffering, a higher dose is therapeutically necessary rather than a sign of the drug-seeking behavior of an addict. At least

five large epidemologic studies have not found benzodiazepine dependence or abuse to be common among those
who are not addicts.

The myth of benzodiazepine dependence and withdrawal
seems to resist all evidence against it. If there is no dependence and withdrawal effects from the sudden cessation of
chronic, high-dose psychoactive medication of any kind, then
I challenge anyone to name the drug. High doses of long-
standing medications of any kind, whether psychiatric or
medical, should never be cut cold turkey, but instead gradually tapered and withdrawn.

The Impending Revival of the
Old Antianxiety and Hypnotic Drugs

I detect the same receptor subdivision strategy about to be
employed on benzodiazepines as was used with the antidepressants. All eleven of the new antidepressants listed in this volume
are variants of norepinephrine, serotonin, and to a slight
extent, dopamine, and are descendents of the old tricyclics
Tofranil and Elavil. The biochemists are beginning the same
dissection of the anxiety receptor. This is the benzodiazepine-
sensitive GABA-A receptor, of which there are now at least
three subunits. One author describes a dozen subunits. New
drugs are being developed to target these subunits, which
allegedly possess no sedative hypnotic or amnestic action. All
the sins of the old benzodiazepines, many of which they are,
in fact, not guilty, are about to be dissolved by the biochemists
and the marketing arms of the drug companies. In the case
of the new antidepressants, this strategy had some value.
Although it did not cure depression, it solved the side effect
and danger in overdose problem so that the drugs could be
more widely administered safely and could help more people.
The benzodiazepine issue is much less compelling. These drugs
are safe in overdose, and are widely and effectively employed in
medical and psychiatric practices around the country. The first

products of this strategy are already available—Sonata and Ambien—which may have some advantage over their predecessors, although others debate this, but I suspect many more will come. This will cost millions of dollars of short in-supply healthcare dollars for what I am afraid will be little added value.

Summary

If you can't sleep no matter what you have done, a benzodiazepine, or one of its refined descendants, will help you for as long as necessary with little or no harm.

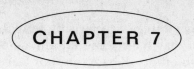

CHAPTER 7

What If You're Still Depressed?

The new drugs make most depressed people feel like their old selves, and some who have been down for years feel better than they can ever remember. In this spirit of excitement and the hope that effective, safe relief from this painful affliction is now available, I am reluctant to temper enthusiasm with talk of failure. It is tempting to promise, as the ad in the psychiatric journals does, that Prozac will "restore the person within the patient," and much more dreary to add the qualifier that this is true in only 50 percent of cases. It is important that you know that if the initial treatment does not work for you or your loved one (although the chances are very good that it will), you should not lose hope, because there are many other helpful alternatives available.

You should be prepared for the fact that 40 (some say 50) percent of people fail to respond to the first antidepressant they try, whether it is an SSRI or any other. Of this group, half do not respond because the medication does not work, and the other half because of an inability to tolerate the side effects. This means that when and if you decide to begin antidepressant medication, you should do so with the hope that you will be helped, but not necessarily by the first drug. Rather than thinking there is one miracle drug that will cure you, it is better to have the attitude that there are a group of outstanding medications, one of which has a great chance of being effective, though which one that is may not be evident on the first try.

If you are able to tolerate the side effects of the first drug and have not responded fully after a month at full dosage, it makes sense to take stock of the following factors when deciding what to do:

1. If you feel a little better, then allow more time, and perhaps try a higher dosage (especially if it is a non-SSRI with a higher cure rate at bigger amounts). You probably will need another month or two on the same drug if you are able to stand the pain and can wait. Those with very severe symptoms may not have that luxury.
2. If you are severely ill, then it may take as much as six months before you feel normal on any drug. You should try to be patient until the medication works fully.
3. If you have not responded in the least at full dosage after several months, it is time to taper off the drug you are on (it is rarely advisable to stop suddenly) and prepare to go on another.

Trying Again

If you don't respond to the first drug tried or cannot tolerate it, it is advisable to try a second one. These days, most people receive an SSRI first. Many who stop because of side effects respond comfortably to a second SSRI. But those who can tolerate but do not get better on full dosage of a first SSRI may want to switch to a different kind of antidepressant. There haven't been any carefully controlled studies to determine whether a drug of a different family is more effective than another SSRI, but clinical lore favors Wellbutrin, Effexor, Serzone, and perhaps Remeron or Cymbalta over a second SSRI. I know of individual cases in which a person responded to a second SSRI, and others where the non-SSRI worked. In any event, about half of the initial 40 to 50 percent of drug failures respond to the second drug. By this time, about 80 percent have significantly improved, although they may not be entirely well.

There are several groups of patients that seem to respond less well to the first drug tried. Elderly people can be less responsive, as can those with very severe symptoms, those with psychotic or bipolar depression, and those who have other psychiatric or medical conditions complicating their depression. Before embarking on rising doses, changing drugs, or combining them in all sorts of innovative ways, attention must be paid to why you did not respond. Do you have something other than a simple depression, such as an unsuspected medical illness or life circumstances that need to be altered? Are you taking a drug that is depressing you? Are you drinking too much alcohol? Is your personality defeating your efforts to enjoy life? In most clinical trials, these complicated cases are excluded when a new antidepressant is tested. Thus, research subjects are usually fairly young (in their thirties and forties), do not have other psychiatric or medical illnesses, are not chronically depressed or suicidal, and are not taking other drugs. Once the FDA approves the medication, it is prescribed for the difficult, previously unresponsive person on whom it was never tried. The difference between the "easy" conditions for which the drug was originally given and the "hard" ones it must combat in the real world can easily be seen if one observes the placebo response in the prerelease subject and in the real one. In the former, it is 25 to 40 percent, whereas in the treatment-resistant patient, it is 0 to 10 percent. It takes a powerful drug to improve or cure treatment-resistant depression, not a sugar pill.

Treatment-Resistant Depression (TRD)

Twenty percent of people fail to improve on either the first or second drug tried. These people are called treatment resistant. At this point, there are two options: adding another drug to the existing treatment or changing to a third drug. While there is no convincing evidence indicating whether switching is better than adding, it seems sensible to switch in order to avoid drug interactions and the increased expense of two medicines at once. If, for example, Paxil failed first and Wellbutrin second, then try a third antidepressant or add one of the following drugs to Wellbutrin:

Lithium
Thyroid (T₃)
A tricyclic
A stimulant
A second new antipressant

If these alternatives (to be discussed in the following sections) fail, it is possible to turn at any time to the still most effective treatment of depression: electroshock therapy (see page 210).

The less proven second drug additions, which have no controlled but only anecdotal support, are:

Reserpine
Antipsychotic drugs
A high-dose MAOI
A tricyclic-and-MAOI combination
Yohimbine
An anticonvulsant
L-tryptophan
Estrogen
Buspirone

Adding Lithium

Lithium is a naturally occurring substance that is primarily used in treating manic-depressive illness. The addition of 600 to 900 mg per day of lithium is the best studied next step against TRD. Some people get better rapidly and dramatically, and others more slowly when lithium is added. The Prozac/lithium combination can be troubled by unpleasant side effects. After four weeks, over 50 percent of TRD patients improve following the addition of lithium, although the initial enthusiasm for lithium addition has waned because it is not as effective as first thought, has many side effects, requires periodic blood checks, and can be lethal in overdose.

Adding Thyroid (T3)

L-triiodothyronine (T3) is produced by the thyroid. It can also be administered in the form of a drug (Cytomel). Added to the previously ineffective antidepressant, T3 speeds the response. Patients with even mild thyroid abnormalities, women over fifty, and depessed people whose muscular movements are slowed seem to do best on thyroid augmentation. It is generally thought that 25 to 50 percent of tricyclic-treated TRD patients improve when T3 is added, and there is little toxicity risk in doing so.

Combining a Tricyclic with an SSRI

Combination of the tricyclic desipramine with Prozac or some other SSRI seems to work well, but needs further controlled proof of its effectiveness. When Prozac or Paxil is the first drug tried, it must be remembered to keep the desipramine doses small (e.g., 50 mg) because of the effect of these two SSRIs on liver metabolism, raising the tricyclic blood level, while Zoloft presents less of an interaction worry.

Adding Ritalin or Dexedrine

Ritalin and Dexedrine are stimulants, and as such, may increase the energy and decrease the lethargy of some depressed patients. There is no controlled research to support the practice of adding them to antidepressants, but one open study found that five of seven TRD patients improved rapidly and markedly with this combination. Pemoline (Cylert), another stimulant, can also be added instead of Ritalin or Dexedrine, and is easier to prescribe because it is not a class II controlled substance, and as such can be called in by the doctor to the pharmacist over the phone. However, because Cylert has been associated with life-threatening liver failure, I would recommend against its use for TRD.

In my experience, an occasional TRD patient responds dramatically to the addition of up to 30 mg of Dexedrine or up to 60 mg of Ritalin without suffering side effects or ending up abusing the drug. People who drink a lot of coffee may do better, whereas those who cannot tolerate caffeine may not like a stimulant drug, but this is not an infallible predictor. Since it is not possible to know in advance who will benefit from the addition of a stimulant, it is worth a trial in the suffering TRD person.

People with TRD vary in their response to stimulants, from those who feel agitated and "wired," to those who initially feel better and then show no signs of improvement, to still others who respond well to a low dose and continue to do so for months or even years.

Provigil (Modafinil)

In doses of 200 to 400 mg in the morning, Provigil produces wakefulness by an unknown mechanism. Because it is believed to lack addiction potential, none of the controlled substance restrictions placed on Dexedrine and Ritalin are in force. This means it can be prescribed in quantities without specific limit, is refillable one to five times within six months

of the original prescription date, and the physician may prescribe it over the telephone. Ritalin and Dexedrine prescriptions must be in writing, may only be prescribed in thirty-day
quantities, and are nonrefillable.

The FDA has restricted Provigil's use to improving wakefulness in patients with excessive daytime sleepiness due to nar-
colepsy, prolonged inability to adjust to shift work, and sleep
apnea. The maker of Provigil had sought approval in all cases
of fatigue and daytime weariness, but was refused. Once a
drug is legally approved, physicians are permitted to prescribe it for whatever conditions they deem reasonable. Thus,
it didn't take long before it was tried for fatigue and sleepiness due to antidepressant side effects, to depression itself, to
augment antidepressants in treatment-resistant patients, in
ADHD, and in fibromyalgia.

The drug does not interfere with nighttime sleep and the
most common side effects are headache and nervousness. In
general, Provigil is well tolerated.

Strattera (Atomoxetine)

As a nonstimulant, Stattera also dodges the controlled substance restrictions put on Dexedrine and Ritalin. As a selective
norepinephrine reuptake inhibitor (SNRI), it is more effective
than placebo in ADHD, but has not been directly compared to methylphenidate (Ritalin, Ritalin-SR, Metadate ER,
Metadate CD, Concerta) or to Adderall or Adderall-XR
(amphetamine/dextroamphetamine).

Atomoxetine has antidepressant properties as well, but
since the SNRI Vestra (reboxetine) has been held up because
of insufficient antidepressant efficacy, it may be that Eli Lilly
decided to go with Strattera for ADHD alone. It comes in doses
of 5-, 10-, 18-, 25-, 40-, and 60-mg capsules. Because it is also
used in children, its dosage is calculated as 1 to 1.2 mg/kg/d.
In adults, it is started at 40 mg per day and after three days
increased to 80 mg per day. It is administered either as a

single dose in the morning or as divided ⬛
and early evening.

Sleep disturbances, dry mouth, problems ur⬛
dizziness, and sexual problems are the most c⬛
effects. Since this is a new drug, even though it has ⬛
tage of presumably lacking abuse potential, it must be ⬛
bered that stimulants have been used safely by million⬛
patients for a long period of time, and remain the treatme⬛
of choice for ADHD.

Combining Antidepressants

The theory behind these combinations of new antidepressants for TRD patients is the attempt to stimulate several
neurotransmitters at once: serotonin, norepinephrine, and
dopamine. While there is no controlled data to prove this
strategy efficacious, it is nonetheless commonly employed:

Remeron + Effexor
Remeron + SSRI
Remeron + Wellbutrin
Effexor + Wellbutrin
Effexor + SSRI
Serzone + Wellbutrin
SSRI + Wellbutrin

For the 10 to 15 percent who remain ill even after combinations of an antidepressant with lithium, thyroid, a tricyclic, a
stimulant, or a second new antidepressant, who are suffering
and deeply discouraged, having difficulty working, and are
a burden to themselves and their families, whose distress is
severe and danger of suicide great, electroshock therapy should
be considered.

Therapy
Therapy, or ECT)

doses in the morning

nating, nausea,
ommon side
he advan-
cemem-
s of
it

a hangover, you realize how
on. In severe depression, the
werful, whether they are due
e ancients thought, to "black
he misery of depression lasts
y certain depressions occur,
ning our sleep, our ability to
nterest in food, sex, and hob-
bies. Depression can also destroy our feelings of love and friendship, rob us of laughter, cause us to turn to alcohol for anesthesia, and make us feel completely alone in our misery. Furthermore, the reason for all this suffering may remain unknown, or the reasons offered by the patient or a family member may seem too trivial to be judged causal.

Psychiatrists would like to be able to point to verifiable causes of clearly defined diseases, but instead must list symptoms occurring together comprising syndromes which give the picture of illnesses, but whose origin is unknown. Electroshock therapy is a treatment in which a current of electricity is passed through the brain. It is not known exactly how or why it works to relieve depression, but it has been shown to be effective when all other treatments have failed. At first, the alternative of ECT may seem barbaric to the patient and concerned loved ones around him or her, and even to the physician, who may wonder whether he or she is reacting out of frustration at being unable to cure what can be an annoying, complaining person or a stoic who denies that anything is wrong, when so much obviously is. Perhaps the physician should try harder to understand, to listen more carefully to the patient's account of his or her pain, and to offer relief through empathy, thus sharing the burden of the distress. It is too easy for the helper to avoid the sufferer's need for a touch of humanity and turn out of haste and avoidance to the magic of electricity. There are bad doctors who have run "shock factories" in which ECT was given routinely, without thought or caring. But there are other kinds of bad doctors and therapists who wait too long while continuing ineffective psychotherapy and drugs for those in severe pain, 15 percent of whom commit suicide. The patient may reject help and maintain a falsely brave front while secretly preparing to terminate his life. The physician may have to urge, even force, electroshock on reluctant or resistant individuals who fear their brains will be fried and damaged and their memories destroyed. Some disturbed psychiatric patients are like people in a coma, in need of emergency treatment without being aware of it, and unless someone takes responsibility (the next of kin or legal conservator), such a person could commit suicide or die from starvation.

Modern ECT is not medieval torture or a form of barbarism. The anesthetist administers a muscle relaxant and oxygen, and puts the patient to sleep, allaying the fears of both the recipient and his or her relatives. Overall, dramatic relief occurs in over 80 percent of those treated, and in about 50 to 75 percent of the TRD patients. Those who have been helped by it return requesting ECT again when and if their depression recurs. They are often unwilling to wait for what they consider useless drug and psychotherapy trials, and want relief as rapidly as possible. The treatments do not necessarily require the patient to be hospitalized, only someone to drive them home afterward, and sometimes can be done while the person continues in his usual occupation. The electrodes can both be placed over the right cerebral hemisphere for a right-handed person (unilateral nondominant) or on both sides of the head (bilateral). The modern use of unilateral (one-sided) ECT significantly decreases the problem of post-treatment amnesia, although bilateral administration is more effective and should be tried if unilateral ECT does not work.

Memory problems following ECT, whether one-sided or bilateral, are minimal. They are confined, when present, to information acquired shortly before ECT was given. Memory difficulties usually disappear completely within six months of treatment.

ECT is equal to, if not superior to, all other therapies used to treat severe TRD. About 50 to 75 percent of those who do not respond to antidepressants improve with ECT. Once the TRD patient recovers, it is necessary either to use drugs or to continue ECT to prevent recurrence. Some people, unfortunately, do not improve after a full course of twelve ECT treatments (including at least six bilateral ones). Following a brief medication-free period, a previously untried antidepressant drug may be successful, perhaps because the ECT has somehow changed the sensitivity of the synapse.

Why Am I Still Depressed?

If you continue to be depressed after trying an antidepressant, there may be another factor contributing to your condition. These factors are:

Type of depression
Medical illnesses
Drugs causing depression
Complicating psychiatric illnesses
Demographic factors

Type of Depression

Some kinds of depression respond better to certain drugs than others do. The diagnosis of psychotic depression can be missed because the patients are ashamed and hide their delusion (a false fixed belief) that they are worthless and feel utter despair. When they are treated with an antidepressant drug alone, only 35 percent respond, whereas 70 percent of nondelusional depressives recover. When an antipsychotic is added to the antidepressant, there is a much higher recovery rate. If this fails, ECT may be necessary, and is most effective.

Atypical depressives (those whose moods are reactive to the environment and who sleep and eat too much) respond better to MAOIs (Nardil, Parnate) and sometimes to the new antidepressants. Bipolar patients without energy may do better on MAOIs and/or possibly on Wellbutrin and lithium.

Medical Illnesses Interfering with Depression Recovery

The following is a list of medical conditions that can cause depression or interfere with its cure. If you suffer from any of these, be sure to let your doctor know before an anti-depressant is prescribed.

Anemia
Gastrointestinal disease (e.g., Crohn's disease)
Neurological diseases
   multiple sclerosis
   Parkinson's disease
   Huntington's disease
   dementia
   stroke
   brain tumors
Endocrine diseases
   thyroid
   pituitary
   adrenal
Infectious diseases
   hepatitis
   influenza
   AIDS
Lupus erythematosus
Heart disease
Malignancies

Drugs That Cause or Worsen Depression

Many drugs used to treat medical conditions may cause or worsen depression, making it more difficult to cure. If you are taking any of the following drugs, be sure to let your physician know before an antidepressant is prescribed.

Drugs for high blood pressure
   Inderal (propranolol)
   Catapres (clonidine)
   Aldomet (methyldopa)
   reserpine
Cortisone
Hormones
   estrogen
   progesterone
Anticancer drugs
   vincristine
   vinblastine
Parkinson's disease drugs
   Sinemet, etc. (levodopa, carbidopa)
   amantadine

Simultaneous Psychiatric Conditions Making Recovery More Difficult

If the factors just cited can be ruled out, then other psychiatric or personality disorders should be considered as reasons for why antidepressant drug therapy has failed. These so-called comorbid states (the simultaneous appearance of two or more illnesses, like depression and alcoholism, in which one may be causing the other, or both may be the product of some hidden factor) are evidence of the difficulty in clearly delineating psychiatric conditions. The hospital chart of a chronic patient almost never lists one pure illness, but a large number of psychiatric and personality disorders. Here are some of the disorders that impede recovery from depression:

Double Depression
People with lifelong dysthymia (chronic low-grade depression) are subject to superimposed major depressions, and

after treatment may not fully recover but return to their chronic dysthymia.

Obsessive-Compulsive Disorder (OCD)

Sufferers of OCD also have frequent major depressive episodes. An antidepressant may relieve their depression, but not their OCD. OCD patients need higher doses of serotonergic antidepressants for many months in order for their OCD to improve. Unfortunately, many, while significantly helped, do not completely recover.

Panic Disorder

Panic disorder patients are prone to episodes of major depression, and major depressives are prone to panic attacks. A person with panic disorder who develops major depression recovers more slowly than someone with depression alone, and has a poorer response to antidepressants. Major depressives who are very anxious but do not suffer panic attacks are also slower in their response to medication. This does not mean you should be overly concerned about your panic disorder, but you should be prepared to wait a little longer until your antidepressant works.

Alcohol and Substance Abuse

More than a quarter of all depressives abuse alcohol or illicit drugs. Ongoing substance abuse in depressed people spoils their response to antidepressant medication. The alcohol or drug problem must be addressed separately and successfully controlled in order for the depression to be medicated and resolved.

Two self-administered tests for alcoholism are widely used: the CAGE and the MAST. The term CAGE refers to a device used to remember four questions: (1) Have you ever had to *c*ut down on alcohol? (2) Has anyone *a*nnoyed you with descriptions of how much you drink? (3) Have you felt *g*uilty about the quantity you consume? (4) Have you needed an *e*ye-opener to get going or relieve a hangover? The Michigan Alcoholism Screening Test (MAST) includes twenty-five items consisting of questions about the amount of drinking and alcohol-related, next-day memory loss, family complaints, fights, work interference, liver cirrhosis, DTs (delirium tremens), hospitalizations, and about morning drinking, drunk driving, and alcohol-related arrests.

When new antidepressant drugs are studied before FDA approval, they are tried on people who are *not* active substance abusers. The reason is that antidepressant drug failures are high among alcoholics and drug addicts. In one study of bipolar disorder, there were five times as many treatment failures in the abuse group as in the nonabuse group. If alcohol or drugs have made you depressed, or if you take them because you are depressed, you need to stop this self-injurious behavior in order for your antidepressant drug to work.

Eating Disorders

People with bulimia or anorexia nervosa and major depression do not respond very well to antidepressants alone, and require a combination of behavior therapy, group therapy, and nutritional guidance.

Personality Disorders

Personality disorders are defined by the *Diagnostic and Statistical Manual of Mental Disorders* (4th ed., 1994) as patterns of inflexible and maladaptive traits that cause subjective distress and significant impairment in social life and occupational functioning. These patterns are continually present since childhood or adolescence and influence

- awareness, perception, reasoning, and judgment
- the regulation of emotions
- control over impulses
- how needs are gratified
- how the person relates to others

People with personality disorders are inflexible, respond poorly to the changes and demands of life, and lack resilience. Most of them are unaware that their personality causes them problems, deny they have difficulties, and are quick to blame others. People with personality disorders have trouble with all aspects of their lives; they are likely to have stormy relationships, to be divorced, and to be fired from jobs. These adversities in their work, social, and intimate lives make them vulnerable to depression, and impede their recovery once they become ill.

There are three schools of thought about the relationship between personality disorder and depression: (1) Certain kinds of personalities lead to depression; (2) Suffering from depression changes personality; and (3) Personality and depression are both influenced by the same underlying genetic forces. There are ten personality disorders listed in the *DSM* IV:

The Odd Cluster	The Dramatic, Emotional, Erratic Cluster	The Anxious, Fearful Cluster
Paranoid	Antisocial	Avoidant
Schizoid	Borderline	Dependent
Schizotypal	Histrionic	Obsessive-
	Narcissistic	Compulsive

While depressive symptoms can occur in anyone with a personality disorder, they are most common in the dramatic and anxious clusters. The dramatic group are impulsive, their inhibitions toward action lowered, and their moods unstable, rapidly shifting in response to frustration or separation from the people who are important to them. Fifty percent of those with borderline personality disorder suffer significant depression, which does not respond well to antidepressant drugs. Borderline persons feel empty, lonely, needy, and angry. They are supersensitive to rejection, have stormy or nonexistent interpersonal relationships, and are subject to moods that are reactive, indeed too reactive, to the environment. SSRIs help borderlines, but more proof of their efficacy in treating this condition is needed. Long-term psychotherapy is essential in this group of individuals.

Assertive, independent, competitive people are more likely to respond to antidepressant drug treatment than are those who are dependent and seek the fulfillment of their needs through other people. Perhaps the latter group would do better on long-term psychotherapy.

A depressed person with medical, psychiatric, and personality complications can be helped by antidepressant medication, but the cure becomes more difficult. The other factors must be addressed and modified to aid the antidepressant in its therapeutic effect. The Greek philosopher Heraclitus said in the fifth century B.C. that "a man's character is his fate." If his character keeps destroying his family, intimacies, and work life, and leaves him vulnerable to depression, then the pill alone is not the answer.

Demographics of Depression

Demography is the study of the characteristics of a certain population. Nowhere is this study trickier than in depression, in which it is necessary to differentiate personality features and the severity and duration of the illness from factors such as age, sex, education, income, social supports, and marital and work status which seem to predict outcome. These factors, so-called demographics, can be nothing more than measurements of the severity and chronicity of the illness. For example, a chronically, seriously ill depressed woman has less energy and confidence to go out and meet men, and therefore is more likely to remain single. To say she is depressed because she is unmarried makes no sense. A person may be sick because of being unmarried or because of marital difficulty, or the individual may be single or in a bad marriage because of being sick. The psychiatric epidemiologist Myrna Weissman found a sixfold increase in marital and family trouble in major depressives. Another study found that women in unhappy marriages had a poorer prognosis for recovery from depression. Is this because depressed people do not get along well with their spouses and are unable to confide in them? While it may be difficult to determine whether the depression caused the marital discord or vice versa, it is clear that working to repair the marital relationship aids the depressed person. Drs. K. Daniel O'Leary and Steven Beach successfully treated thirty-six troubled marriages in which the wives were depressed, resulting in greater marital satisfaction and a significant reduction in depression. Sometimes the marital improvement follows upon the relief of depression rather than causes it. Karen, the forty-year-old married mother of one I mentioned in a previous chapter, whose husband was cold and angry at what he thought to be her laziness and lack of attention to him and their child, became much warmer when Prozac lifted her depression, helping her to get out of bed and look as though she liked, rather than hated, him. Karen's demographics improved because her depression got better.

As bad as marriage can be, depression has been found in epidemiological studies to be much higher among the non-married population. The onset of depression is most likely in single women. Divorce or separation increases the likelihood of a first depressive episode, and decreases the recovery rate once it occurs. But a person's marital status does not affect his or her response to antidepressant drugs.

A depressive is more likely to recover if friends and family are warm, loving, and supportive, and less so if they are critical and hostile. The problem is that sicker depressives frustrate their families more, making them angry and disparaging, while healthier ones are less annoying. Ironically, the more needy the patient, the more the loved ones are turned off. It is the doctor's role to help the critical spouse and angry family to deal with the depressed person in a kinder, more supportive manner, because no matter how powerful the antidepressant medication, it is usually too weak to work all by itself, and requires the help of a friendly family.

Paula Clayton, of Washington University in St. Louis, and

her colleagues found that a close, confiding relationship and physical closeness protected people from depression. Other investigators have discovered that the absence of social supports increases the patient's vulnerability to depression. Since depression keeps people home, withdrawn from society, this may be simply one more measurement of severity. People too impaired to go out and build and maintain social supports may become depressed because they are too sick to socialize, making the finding a redundancy. It does no good to suggest to the depressed that they venture out and form meaningful relationships so they will feel better.

Negative life events decrease the rate of recovery on antidepressant drugs. While this seems obvious, it pays to remember that if you lose your job or your lover or develop a serious medical illness while being treated with Prozac for depression, your recovery will be slowed down.

Summary: Steps to Take If You or a Loved One Are Treatment Resistant

1. Take an antidepressant that agrees with you (i.e., the side effects are bearable) for several months at the right dose. If there is some noticeable improvement, give it more time, perhaps six months or a year, until you fully recover. But if after several months you feel no better, taper off and then stop.

2. The second drug you take may, but probably should not, belong to the same class as the first. Follow an SSRI with Wellbutrin, Serzone, Effexor, Remeron, Cymbalta, or a tricyclic.

3. If you remain symptomatic, ask your doctor to add lithium, thyroid, a tricyclic antidepressant, or a stimulant to the antidepressant you are currently taking.

4. If everything up to now has failed, and you or a loved one remains in severe pain and unable to function for over a year, a course of twelve ECT treatments (six bilateral ones) should be considered before more time elapses and the

suffering, despair, and suicidal thoughts worsen. This seemingly barbaric treatment has been modernized and civilized, and can produce startling results in the carefully chosen person.

5. If you and your doctor decide to skip the ECT step because you are adamantly opposed to it or not incapacitated enough, there are a series of other drugs you can try whose efficacy has mostly anecdotal support, and sometimes a smattering of controlled, objective verification. They are:

Reserpine
Antipsychotics
An MAOI
An MAOI-tricyclic combination
An anticonvulsant
L-tryptophan
Estrogen
Buspirone
Yohimbine

6. If you still continue to be depressed, review the original diagnosis carefully, making sure of the following: you do not have previously unsuspected psychotic depression; there is no unknown medical condition preventing recovery; other drugs you are taking are not making you depressed; and you do not have a simultaneous psychiatric illness or personality disorder preventing recovery.

The End of Depression

Depressed people experience their demographics as bad, and must convert the most important of them to good—working alone, in a support group, or with a friend, therapist, or member of the clergy.

Demographics, as I have defined them before, are the characteristics describing a group of people: their age, sex, education, marital status, occupation, income level, family size, community involvement, religious affiliation, leisure pursuits, etc. Think about these parts of your life and how you would rate them. Depressed people usually regard their demographics as miserable. The depressive's demographics are experienced as: age—too old; sex—the wrong one; education—defective; marriage—miserable; single—hopelessly so; job—unbearable; income—inadequate; family—childless, none, or too demanding; community involvement—none or too much; religion—none or dissatisfied with; and leisure activities—boring. Direct work on the demographics of the TRD's (treatment-resistant depressive's) life is absolutely necessary and can be very helpful. Somewhere in this list often lies the most important part of the depressive's life, which makes the rest unacceptable and is the reason why the person is resistant to all antidepressants, whether old, new, or yet to be released. If marital therapy can make some people less depressed, as has been shown, then finding out what an individual's most important issue is and helping him or her to change it from miserable to pleasurable can result in startling improvement. A partially working antidepressant can sometimes provide enough help so that the person can overcome that which has kept him or her depressed, but it is the demographic change which will convert the half-improved depressive to a cured one.

I remember several questions, all referring to this essential point of change from depression to a life of energy and pleasure, posed by two men of very different, yet similar occupations, for whom I have the greatest respect: the late Elvin Semrad, M.D., psychiatrist, psychoanalyst, and teacher, and Father John Padberg, S.J. Semrad's questions were asked of patients interviewed in front of psychiatrists in training, and Father John's were asked of me alone late one evening. These words may not make the most exciting reading, but pause and try to honestly answer them. Believe me, they are not easy.

What do you really care about?
Whom do you really care about?

What do you need to do for yourself to make your life better?
Why are you not doing it?

These questions do not allow the avoidance maneuver of the personality disorder sufferer, who blames his or her woes on others. Fix what you can fix and learn to accept and make the best of what you cannot. Go back and read the depressive demographics; make the best of those you cannot change and radically alter those you can. Do it alone or work with a therapist or someone else you trust, but start the job today of fixing your life for the better. It seems obvious to me that if after all the steps described in this chapter, you are still not cured, then the cure is meant to come not from outside people or medications but from within. Ask yourself what you need so as not to be depressed, and go get it.

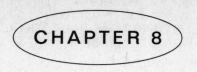

CHAPTER 8

Herbal Medicines

A standing-room-only audience at the American Psychiatric Association in 1998 listened to experts from the National Institute of Mental Health, the UCLA Department of Psychiatry, and others describe the benefits and possible hazards of herbal medicines. The establishment was being forced to take notice of the populace, their patients. Since 1962 the FDA, under the Kefauver-Harris drug amendments, passed because of Thalidomide-induced birth deformities, has been protecting the population by making sure that drugs are safe and efficacious. The FDA approves all clinical testing plans and makes sure of the competence of investigators. It also supervises the safety and efficacy of over-the-counter products. Under the eye of the government, pharmaceutical companies develop new antidepressant drugs and physicians dispense them. The patient is being protected.

In democratic countries, the populace does not remain docile while the government oversees their safety, especially since the antidepressant drugs, while having been made less toxic and safer when overdoses are taken, have not improved the cure rate of depression in over forty years. I have questioned many leading psychopharmacologists, who agree with me that as a result of antidepressant treatment, 30 percent fully recover, another 35 percent partially improve, and 35 percent remain ill.

There are a number of reasons for the growth in alternative methods for the treatment of depression. There is the embarrassment and expense of having to see a doctor to get medicine. A busy family physician may allot merely five minutes of talk about the problem, which can feel like lack of interest. A number of us wish to control our own medication. In the case of herbal products, many people desire to take a natural substance.

The interest in alternative therapies is stimulating drug companies and the FDA to respond to the consumer. In 1994 Congress passed the Dietary Supplement Health and Education Act, which allows manufacturers to advertise the health effects of herbal supplements without having to scientifically prove their claims or assure their safety because they are classified as neither foods nor drugs. The major pharmaceutical houses like American Home Products (under the name Centrum), Bayer, Merck, and others are beginning to market herbal products with the stamp of purity and safety associated with their respected companies. Unfortunately, brand names alone are not a guarantee of good science, safety, purity, and efficacy. Less scrupulous companies can make false claims as cure-alls, their products can be dangerous rather than safe, and there is no assurance the package contains what the label says, especially if the herb is scarce or expensive.

Part of the issue is political and philosophical. How much do we trust and want government to look after our safety at the cost of individual freedom, and how much do we want to be left alone to take whatever herb or tonic we wish? The pharmaceutical houses would be happy to have FDA regulators off their backs. Since it costs more than 250 million dollars to introduce a new antidepressant under federal guidelines, it would be much cheaper to put some St. John's Wort in clean bottles and let the government-funded NIMH do the research to prove its safety and efficacy. The companies might even be willing to pass along the savings to the customers. The herbs would be cheaper and the expense of doctor visits spared. Then again, if the government has to pay for the research, the consumer's saving might be diminished by the need for higher taxes.

To summarize, there are pros and cons to herbal medicines. The pros are that they are cheaper and easily available; you do not have to reveal your problems to a doctor who often doesn't know you, or be forced to sit through a lecture by a physician about the danger of addiction in order to get them. Thus control would be put back in the public's hands. The cons are that relaxation of current regulatory practices of herbal drugs could lead to ineffective agents being used in potentially lethal conditions such as serious depression; doctors would not be consulted and thus miss the chance to diagnose and treat physical and psychological causes of depression. In addition, inadequately researched and perhaps ineffective herbal remedies for milder depression can allow the damage to the confidence, career, social, and family life of the sufferer to go unchecked. The treatment of the devastating disorder of depression should not be relegated to snake oil.

David A. Kessler, then head of the FDA (now dean of Yale University's Medical School), unsuccessfully fought the 1994 law that weakened the agency's authority to regulate herbal medicines for fear people with serious conditions would be attracted to ineffective treatments. In the July 23, 1998, *New York Times* he stated, "If you promote a product as a Mood Minder, you have a responsibility to that person who is depressed, and if that product doesn't work, you are doing harm." Ephedra, for example, which provides an amphetamine-like rush, weight loss, and perhaps increased sexual pleasure can also cause heart attacks, strokes, and seizures.

The common assumption that if a product is natural, an herb, it must be safe is incorrect. A 1996 article in the *Annals of Internal Medicine*, entitled "Coma from the Health Food Store: Interaction Between Kava and Alprazolam (Xanax)," emphasizes that point. Plants can be poisonous and even kill. The flower digitalis, for example, can have therapeutic effects on the heart. If an overdose is taken, though, it can cause fatalities.

The debate between those who would allow people more freedom and those who would protect people from themselves is a fierce one. One side depicts the government, the doctors, and the drug companies in a giant conspiracy against freedom, while the other sees them as protecting innocent consumers.

There is a further move on to liberalize the regulation of not only herbal medicines but prescription drugs themselves. Some argue that these agents should be controlled for a limited number of years until deemed safe and effective and then be sold over-the-counter. They claim it hard to imagine what harm could now come from Prozac becoming available without a doctor's order.

I believe more freedom for people is warranted. If we allow them to have cars and guns, the potential damage from St. John's Wort, kava, or even Prozac seems pale by comparison. If the government permits cigarettes and whiskey, how much damage can herbs or psychiatric drugs do?

St. John's Wort (*Hypericum perforatum*)

Hypericum is the extract from the flower of St. John's Wort, and this herb has been used for hundreds of years to treat anxiety and insomnia. It has been given in purified form and in whole-plant preparation. Psychopharmacologists favor isolating pure compounds and determining their effects on specific receptors, while ethnic herbalists believe therapeutic power is strengthened by administering the whole plant and only diluted by reducing it to hypericin, which is the most toxic part of the plant and may not be the only active constituent. In the United States, one-fourth of all prescriptions are derived from just forty plant species. Codeine and morphine come from poppies. The rosy periwinkle provides the anti-cancer drugs Vincristine and Vinblastine. Curare, derived from plants from the Amazon, aids anesthesia. The snakeroot provides reserpine for hypertension. Advanced cancers are treated by Taxol from the bark of the yew, and high fevers from the bark of the willow tree in the form of its main compound salicylate, made in the laboratory into aspirin.

The thirteen trials that compared a single hypericum preparation with placebo reported a 22.3 percent response to the sugar pill versus 55.1 percent for hypericum (St. John's Wort). Since the subjects were mild to moderately depressed out-patients, the placebo response rate seems too low. If it were closer to the 40 or even 50 percent that I would anticipate, St. John's 55.1 percent success would not be statistically superior.

The dosage of St. John's Wort has not been standardized. Typically, people take extracts of 0.3 percent hypercin of which 300 to 900 mg are given per day. This equals two to four grams of the dried herb. There are far fewer side effects than from standard antidepressants. The most common are dry mouth, gastrointestinal symptoms, dizziness, confusion, and fatigue, which occur in less than one percent. There is some question about whether taking the drug increases skin sensitivity to strong sunlight. There appear to be no sexual side effects. No studies of long-term safety exist, and it is not recommended for use in pregnancy and lactation. The mechanism of its antidepressant action is unknown. Some believe St. John's Wort inhibits the reuptake of serotonins, norepinephrine, and dopamine as well as acting on the same gamma-aminobutyric acid (GABA) receptors as do the benzodiazepine drugs like Valium and Xanax. It takes twenty-four hours for a half dose to be eliminated from the body. Oddly, it is not known whether the purified extract of St. John's Wort, hypericum, crosses the blood-brain barrier. According to Jack Gorman,

M.D., a research psychiatrist at Columbia University's College of Physicians and Surgeons, the hypericin molecule is too large to cross the blood-brain barrier, which, if true, would make it hard to understand how hypericin could be the active ingredient in St. John's Wort or if the herb is effective at all.

St. John's Wort costs about one-sixth the price of a standard antidepressant. A hundred 375-mg capsules sell for ten to fourteen dollars.

Because there are so many questions about dosage, safety, and efficacy of St. John's Wort, the National Institute of Mental Health (NIMH) completed a study of 336 patients comparing it to 100 mg per day of Zoloft and placebo. Neither Zoloft (sertraline) nor St. John's Wort proved better than placebo (Hypericum Depression Study Group [HDTSG], 2002). In the eight-week, double-blind, randomized comparison of hypericum to placebo and Zoloft, 31.9 percent responded to placebo, 24.8 percent to Zoloft, and 23.9 percent to hypericum. This design shows the importance of a placebo group, or otherwise it would have appeared that St. John's Wort was equal to Zoloft at one-tenth the cost, and with fewer side effects. The vigorous, technical debate about what this all means is beyond the scope of this book. Briefly, it involves study methodology, patient selection, chronicity, depression severity, SSRI effectiveness, potency of placebo, and whether the study site was private or academic. Trial design that emphasizes clinical rather than statistical significance, as well as expert consensus on illness severity and therapeutic outcomes, were recommended.

Two other placebo-controlled studies that did not include an active antidepressant drug, such as Zoloft, split results. Richard Shelton et al. did not find St. John's Wort more effective than placebo in two hundred major depressives in 2001, which critics of the study say are too severely depressed for St. John's Wort to treat, and that Zoloft would have won if higher doses of it had been used in a larger study, since the trend was positive in the drug's favor (*Journal of the American Medical*

Association). In a double-blind, randomized, placebo-controlled trial with 375 patients with mild to moderate depression, a St. John's Wort extract was found to be safe and more effective than placebo by Y. Lecrubier et al. in 2002 (*American Journal of Psychiatry*).

The three studies score one win for St. John's Wort, one loss, and one tie. The world of psychiatric research is very messy, especially when not being run by drug companies.

While I might not take St. John's Wort if I were pregnant, or on other drugs with which it might interact in ways unknown, and certainly not if I were seriously ill, I find it safe and perhaps effective for mild to moderately depressed patients.

Kava

Kava, a beverage made from the roots of the piper methysticum shrub, native to the South Pacific and used there for centuries to provide mild relaxation, is a presumably safe, nonaddicting version of the martini without the hangover. Nonetheless, there are road signs on some Pacific islands warning not to drink kava and drive. In Europe it is taken for anxiety, muscle relaxation, and sedation. In the United States the roots are ground into a powder to be blended into drinks or put into pills or capsules. The pharmacologically active agents in kava include alpha pyrones (also called kavalactones). It may act on the same receptor (GABA) as the benzodiazepines like Valium and Klonopin.

Kava may help tension and anxiety, while allegedly not decreasing mental acuity or coordination. The purity of kava as well as its safety and efficacy have not been established by a single scientific study in human beings in the United States. Clinical trials in Germany and elsewhere have used standardized preparations between 100 and 200 mg of kavalactones daily. Doses over 400 mg for long periods may cause scaling of the skin on the arms and legs, as well as sleepiness and uncoordinatedness, possibly leading to automobile and other accidents. Over one hundred cases of liver damage due to kava use have caused the FDA to issue a warning. It is less potent than drugs like Klonopin and Ativan, and probably ought not to be used.

Valerian

This plant has a mild sedative effect. It is not superior to other hypnotic agents. Two to three grams of the dried root are taken three times daily or at bedtime to induce sleep. It may possibly cause liver damage and is not recommended during pregnancy or nursing, although there are no reports of it causing harm to the newborn.

The following table is modified from an excellent article by Albert H. C. Wong, M.D., et al. (see bibliography).

Black Cohosh

Long used by North American aboriginal peoples to relieve menopausal symptoms, PMS, and painful menstruation, Black cohosh seems to function by suppressing the luteinizing hormone and as an estrogen substitute. A double-blind placebo-controlled study found it superior to placebo for the treatment of the physical and mental symptoms of menopause. The dose used is between 40 and 200 mg daily, and it begins to take effect within two weeks. Its rare side effects include stomach pain and intestinal discomfort. Because no long-term studies exist, it probably should not be taken for more than six months.

German Chamomile

Available as tea or as a liquid extract, it is said to calm anxiety, digestive upset, and help induce sleep. The evidence is not very good, but the product is harmless. If it calms you, use it.

Herbal Remedies Commonly Used to Treat Psychiatric Symptoms

Herb	Common Usage	Quality of Evidence	Adverse Effects	Cautions	Drug Interactions
Black cohosh	Menopause symptoms PMS Dysmenorrhea	+++ + +	Headaches	Pregnancy Lactation	?
German chamomile	Insomnia Anxiety	+ +	Rare	Allergy to sunflower family of plants	0
Evening primrose	Schizophrenia Attention deficit Dementia	0 0 0	None	Mania Epilepsy	Phenothiazines NSAIDs Coricosteroids Beta-blockers Anticoagulants
Ginkgo	Memory loss Concentration difficulties Anxiety Depressed mood	+++ +++ +++ +++	Headache Gastrointestinal upset	Pregnancy Lactation	Anticoagulants
Hops	Insomnia	+	Allergy Menstrual irregularity	Depression Pregnancy Lactation	?
Kava	Insomnia Anxiety Seizures	+ + 0	Scaling of skin on extremities Liver damage Headache	Pregnancy Lactation	Benzodiazopines Alcohol

Herb	Common Usage	Quality of Evidence	Adverse Effects	Cautions	Drug Interactions
Lemon balm	Insomnia Anxiety	o +	None	Thyroid disease Pregnancy Lactation	Central nervous system depressants Thyroid medication
Passion flower	Insomnia Anxiety	+ +	Vasculitis Sedation	Pregnancy Lactation	?
Skullcap	Insomnia Anxiety Seizures	o o o	Sedation Confusion Seizures	Pregnancy Lactation	?
St. John's Wort	Depression	+++	Photosensitivity Gastrointestinal upset Sedation	Cardiovascular disease Pregnancy Lactation Pheochromocytoma	Drugs that interact with MAOI
Valerian	Insomnia Anxiety	+ +	Sedation	Pregnancy Lactation	Central nervous system depressants

Quality of Evidence: +++ acceptable (at least two properly controlled trials)
++ probably acceptable (well supported)
+ expert opinion
o insufficient evidence

Evening Primrose

Recommended by some for the treatment of a large number of disorders, it appears to be worthless but probably also harmless.

Ginkgo

Used widely in Europe, this product of the ginkgo tree (Ginkgo biloba) is used for dementia, memory deficiencies, concentration difficulties, sexual dysfunctioning, anxiety, and depression. It is believed to improve cerebral blood flow. In the form of a standardized extract, 40 mg are taken three times a day for at least three months before the full effect is achieved. Doses up to 360 mg per day are used for treating Alzheimer's disease. A review of eight controlled studies found it to improve memory loss, depressed mood, anxiety, and concentration difficulties. Its primary effectiveness may be on mild memory loss and cerebral circulation, and its effect on anxiety and depression seem secondary. Side effects from ginkgo are uncommon, and include headache, indigestion, and allergic skin reactions.

Hops

The female flowers of the plant used in making beer also have been employed as a mild sedative and sleep aid. There is no evidence supporting its use in insomnia and anxiety disorders. It is given three times daily and at bedtime as 0.5 to 1 gram of dried flowers or 0.5 to 1 milliliter of liquid extract. It should not be given during pregnancy or lactation.

Lemon Balm

This member of the mint family is said by some to be useful in anxiety and to induce sleep. It seems to have no effects or side effects.

Passion Flower

The Aztecs used it as a sedative and sleep inducer. There is not enough objective evidence to support whether or not it works. Inflammation of blood vessels has occurred during its use.

Skullcap

Both the roots and aerial parts of this plant have been used as a tranquilizer and anticonvulsant. There is no evidence to prove it is effective. It can cause liver damage and probably should be avoided.

To Use Herbs or Not

St. John's Wort may be useful in depression, yet no herbal treatment is more effective than current conventional drugs. There is a lot of interest in these plant products, whose history in some cases extends back thousands of years. We must learn more about dosage, effectiveness, and possible dangers in taking them alone or in combination with other drugs. For mild symptoms, if they make people feel better, there is probably very little danger. In chronic depression, even when judged not severe, the damage to self-esteem, energy, motivation, hope, and to social, family, and vocational functioning cannot be eradicated by plants. Therapists and effective drugs are still necessary. If anything, we need better therapists specializing in the treatment of the long-term erosion produced by depression, as well as more effective drugs. While herbs seem like a harmless, time-honored escape from modern misery to a simpler time, we must remember that most of man's medicines before the twentieth century did no good, and some of them did harm. Modern science is a big bother. Its advances are slow and costly. We need inventive researchers, not timid, shortsighted synapse tinkerers. Six SSRIs are more than enough. We not only must have new and better drugs, we also need to rethink what medicine can and cannot do. It is very troubling that only 30 percent fully recover with the best antidepressant drugs. I believe that none of the herbs in this chapter provide a better answer, not even St. John's Wort. But I am glad that ethnobotanists are out in ancient rain forests interviewing shamans and native healers and observing their work with their patients. We need all the help we can get. One factor the ethnobotanists notice is that the rain forest healers usually live with their patients and witness their symptoms firsthand. What we may learn is not that herbs are better, but that a doctor cannot understand and treat a patient in fifteen minutes. A nurse told me how she had discovered the importance of close therapeutic involvement with the people she was trying to help. Tired of hospital bureaucracy and of sitting in the ward office doing paperwork, she decided to become a massage therapist. During the forty-five-minute to hour-and-a-half hands-on sessions, she was amazed to find how much her clients told her of their pains and unhappiness. There was no magic in the massage. It was in the talking and listening that the therapeutic encounter took place. Perhaps this is the ultimate ancient secret of herbal medicine.

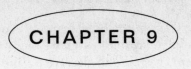

CHAPTER 9

What Does the Future Hold?: Antidepressants Available in Other Places or Being Developed in the United States

When we attend a baseball game, an opera, or a play, the talk often turns to the young talent on the way up. The great ones are easy to spot—unhittable pitchers, blasting batters, soaring singers, enthralling actors. The enjoyment of discovering the new and exciting extends to every area: the latest chef, clothing designer, architect, physician, automobile, computer, presidential candidate. We all yearn for progress and perfection. Nowhere is that yearning stronger than in medicine— the wish to be freed from the misery of painful bodily illness, the horror of cancer and stroke, the broken mind of schizophrenia, and what many describe as the most painful and debilitating affliction of all, depression. Depression both destroys the pleasures of life and makes its inevitable pains completely unbearable. The normal sadness following an illness or death, business reversal, or social slight becomes weighed down by depression, which destroys resilience, the chance for recovery, and the ability to try again.

In this chapter, I will try to be your guide to the antidepressants that are not yet available or that are in development in the United States. Because these drugs are unavailable in the United States and we cannot go and see the production for ourselves, I will be very specific in describing the facts on which I base my reviews of these up-and-coming agents. There are enthusiastic and pessimistic reviewers—those who love the theater, and most of what they see in it, and those with lofty standards met only by John Gielgud and Laurence Olivier. An example of this is the differing views of two distinguished psychiatric professors about the new drugs I am about to describe. Dr. Leo Hollister, of the University of Texas, referred to the pace of development of new psychotherapeutic drugs as "glacial," noting that Prozac and Zoloft, although better tolerated and safer in overdose, are no more effective than antidepressants we have had for the past forty years. Of the new antidepressants in various stages of development, he finds none more effective than those already available. Dr. Carolyn Rabinowitz of George Washington University, on the other hand, is quoted in the July 1994 edition of *Psychiatric Times* on the "marvelous, unprecedented breakthroughs" in effective treatments for mental illness.

How New Drugs Get Released

The Food and Drug Administration is maddeningly slow. A typical drug takes nine years to journey from the beginning of human trials to a pharmacy. Prozac, for example, was created in 1972, clinical trials began in 1976, and the drug was released for marketing in 1988. This is typical. The average time from synthesis of an antidepressant to its release in the United States is fourteen years. Those fond of pointing out how many more drugs are available in Europe denounce our FDA for its excessive bureaucratic procedures, and a few have suggested privatizing the process to protect it from governmental delay. Others say many of the European drugs are marketed without adequate research support, and applaud American thoroughness. While I am sure the FDA could speed up the process without undue risk to the consumer, I also know of no European antidepressant that I would advise hopping on a plane to cross the Atlantic to buy.

There are three ways to find a new antidepressant. One is to give prospective agents to animals who have been placed in experimental environments designed for the screening of antidepressant drugs. A second, employing drug receptors in the brain to identify new compounds, is the most fashionably scientific, but so far has turned up copies of older agents, and no breakthroughs. Finally there is the creativity and intuition of alert, experienced clinicians who have, aided by luck, provided most of the advances in psychopharmacology: lithium, Thorazine, Tofranil, and the MAOIs. Using a new drug in an open trial, astute researchers are able to identify if it is effective, in what dosage, and for which patients. This open, non-blind method has been slighted in recent years in the rush to start formal random controlled trials. More prolonged and leisurely open study would decrease the number of copy-cat drugs and diminish the frequency of expensive, formally researched failures. The rigid, narrowly focused present system leads to antidepressants being released that have never been tried on typical office and hospitalized patients and have not been used long enough to see if they really work.

For every drug that is actually released in the United States, thousands are developed. Of those that are then tried on humans, only a quarter will eventually be approved for sale, after a period averaging about nine years. A new antidepressant will cost about $500 million to bring to market. These high development costs tend to inhibit innovation and provide one explanation for why new SSRIs are constantly being put forward, rather than an antidepressant that is truly novel. Rational drug design can become repetitive design.

Some Antidepressants Unavailable
in the United States

The search is on for antidepressants that are more effective, faster-acting, better tolerated, and safer in overdose than what is currently available. The last of these goals, regarding safety in overdose, seems already to have been achieved by the SSRIs, Serzone, Effexor, Remeron, and Cymbalta. The new drugs are pretty well tolerated, but there is room for improvement in the areas of gastrointestinal upset, agitation, insomnia, and sexual disturbance. But it is in the realm of efficacy and speed of action that the need for improvement is greatest, and in which not much progress has been made in forty years. None of the drugs listed alphabetically in this section, some of which are available outside of the United States, are more effective or faster-acting than those currently available here. You need not lobby your congressional representative to get them released here sooner. What they may provide, however, are different modes of action in fighting depression, and research leads to future breakthroughs. Or perhaps we will have to continue to rely on serendipity. I would encourage doctors to keep their eyes open and not sit back passively in darkened rooms watching the slides of molecular biologists for the answer. I would also encourage their patients to keep telling them what works and what does not, so that the two, doctor and patient, can join in the hunt together. It is a hunt not only for the right drug but for the way to overcome depression, something that in most cases takes much more than a pill.

Some of the descriptions of these drugs will be much longer than others, either because more is known or because the drugs seem to have more promise.

Adinazolam

Available in Europe, this is a benzodiazepine belonging to the same overall family as Valium, and to the same benzodiazepine subfamily as Xanax and Klonopin. In a slow-release preparation, it may be effective in treating panic disorder, but the FDA advisory panel recommended against its approval for this use or for major depression. When taken over time, it apparently sensitizes neurons to serotonin, which may make it worth trying in the treatment of depression. In a four-week trial comparing Elavil, Valium, and Adinazolam in depression, Elavil was best, Valium worst, and Adinazolam in the middle.

Buspar (Buspirone)

Buspirone, gepirone, ipsapirone, tandospirone, and flesi-noxan together constitute a family of drugs known as agonists to the $5HT_{1A}$ receptor. There are at least twelve different subtypes of serotonin receptors located pre- and postsynaptically in the brain and $5HT_{1A}$ is one of them.

Buspirone (Buspar) is available in the United States for the treatment of anxiety. It and several other members of this group of drugs have repeatedly failed tests for antidepressant efficacy. The other members of this class are in various stages of trial, and some may be released here within the next few years. The advantage of Buspar over the benzodiazepines like Valium and Xanax is that it produces very little sedation, abuse, or withdrawal difficulties. Because of its short metabolism, it must be taken three times a day. Unlike the benzodiazepines, Buspar does not produce an immediate effect. In fact, the complete response may take two to four weeks, perhaps because it takes time to desensitize the receptor ($5HT_{1A}$). People who have had benzodiazepines in the past do not like Buspar, because its action is too slow, there is no immediate mild euphoria, and there is no sedating effect. Nervous, anxious people like to be calmed now, not three weeks later. The main side effects of Buspar are headaches, restlessness, insomnia, nausea, and dizziness, a lineup that sounds suspiciously like that of an SSRI. The drug is safe in overdose.

Corticotropin-Releasing Factors (CRF) Antagonists

CRF is the main brain regulator coordinating responses to stress. It acts as a neurotransmitter and as a hormone. Excessive CRF may produce anxiety, sleep and appetite disturbances as well as depression. Several companies are working on drugs blocking CRF excess in the hope they will have antidepressant and antianxiety effects. They may also be useful to combat the stress of traumas, such as rape, as well as before surgery.

Gepirone ER

In extended-release (ER) once-daily form, it is moderately effective in anxiety and major depression. The only side effects are mild dizziness, nausea, insomnia, and gastrointestinal symptoms. It does not seem to cause weight gain, sedation, or sexual side effects. Along with Buspar (buspirone), it acts on a subdivision of the serotonin receptor.

Inositol

This drug is thought to activate intracellularly the receptor of many neurotransmitters. Although it crosses the blood-brain barrier with difficulty, large doses may be effective in treating depression.

Lofepramine

This tricyclic antidepressant is popular in the United Kingdom because it is said to be safe in overdosage and low in side effects. It is superior to a placebo and comparable to other antidepressants. Curiously, its major metabolite is desipramine (Norpramin), a drug we already have plenty of, so I doubt that lofepramine will ever be released here.

Mianserin (Bolvidon, Norval)

This older tetracyclic is probably a little less effective than standard antidepressants, as shown in double-blind studies. In use since 1976, it has never been available in the United States and no one misses it. It is available in five European countries. What interests researchers about mianserin is that it functions a little like Serzone on the serotonin receptor, and a little like idazoxan on the norepinephrine system.

Mifepristone (Mifeprex, RU-486, the Abortion Pill)

Mifepristone is being evaluated for use in the 15 percent of severely depressed patients who are psychotic. These most difficult to treat depressives have delusions, such as of deserving punishment for imagined crimes. The drug, in doses higher than those used to induce abortion, blocks cortisol secreted by the adrenal glands. Cortisol is often elevated in psychotic depression (also see CRF antagonists). It is estimated that at least five more years will be required to establish its effectiveness. If accomplished, the FDA would probably restrict its use, as it did in 2000 when it approved Mifeprex for abortions. Also, since there are other ways to block CRF, unless Mifepristone proves uniquely effective, one that does not induce abortion is likely to prevail in the marketplace.

Minaprine

Minaprine acts on serotonin and dopamine and may be an effective antidepressant. The drug does not seem to be a stimulant or subject to abuse, and its main side effects are insomnia, anxiety, and nausea.

Moclobemide

The conventional MAOIs Nardil and Parnate irreversibly inhibit monoamine oxidase, thus raising the amounts of norepinephrine and serotonin in the synapse. When their use is discontinued, the body requires two weeks before it can produce the natural enzyme monoamine oxidase again. The danger of severe, life-threatening high blood pressure and of the serotonin syndrome (in its worst form producing high fever, circulatory failure, and death) limits the use of these drugs, and requires that careful dietary and medication restrictions be imposed.

The new MAOIs are reversible in their inhibition of monoamine oxidase in the hope that their side effects and dangers, and the dietary restrictions they necessitate, will be much less. Moclobemide is a reversible inhibitor of MAO-A (only the A form is required for antidepressant activity). The class to which it belongs is abbreviated as RIMA (reversible inhibitor monoamine oxidase-A). It is available in Canada and the United Kingdom, and has been used by some investigators for many years. The chance of severe hypertension occurring due to eating certain foods with the drug is reported to be very rare, although caution is advised when combining it with SSRIs or opioids. The dose range is 300 to 900 mg per day.

There are reports that Moclobemide causes irritability, insomnia, anxiety, restlessness, and agitation. Some have found it not to be as effective as Nardil or Parnate. When taken alone in overdose, it is usually not fatal, but causes fatigue, agitation, and high blood pressure. In overdose and combined with other drugs, it can cause coma, high fever, rigidity, and even higher blood pressure, and when overdose of a RIMA is combined with an SSRI or the serotonin tricyclic Anafranil, the result can be lethal. Five deaths from this combination have been reported in Finland. Other RIMA dangers occur when these drugs are mixed with Demerol or nasal decongestants. The picture of the RIMAs continues to sharpen in focus, and does not appear as bright as it once was. Further clinical trials of Moclobemide in the United States have been dropped.

Omega-3 Fatty Acids

One to three grams a day (three to four ounces of salmon or tuna) are supposed to help major depression, bipolar disorder, and aggressive behavior. The two omega-3s that are alleged to be best are DHA and EPA. Since the FDA does not regulate supplements as it does drugs, there is no way to know which brand is best. Consumerlab.com found six of the twenty products did not have the amount of DHA listed on the label. Fish oil can increase the risk of bleeding in people on aspirin or blood thinners. Fishy-smelling breath can be an unpleasant side effect of these agents. I must repeat my usual warning that larger and better studies will be needed to prove whether the claims for omega-3s as an antidepressant are true or not. Several are promised, but so far, none are available.

Ondansetron (Zofran)

This drug affects serotonin and is currently available in the United States as an antiemetic agent for those undergoing chemotherapy, and to prevent postoperative nausea. Animal and human studies suggest that it may possess antianxiety, antidepressive, antipsychotic, antipanic, and anti–social phobic effects.

Prozac II

Eli Lilly joined with another company, Sepracor, to produce Prozac II. Prozac II is an isomer of Prozac I. Isomers are identical molecules whose atoms are arranged as mirror images of one another. One isomer of a drug may produce most of its activity, and the other, its side effects. Unfortunately, R-fluoxetine produced a negative cardiac side effect, and plans for its development were abandoned.

Ritanserin (Tisterton)

This drug has serotonin action similar to that of Serzone ($5HT_{1A}$ antagonist) and mianserin, and has promise of being an effective antidepressant. It is said to work in dysthymic and anxiety disorder patients as well. The drug is fairly far along in American clinical trials for other psychiatric disorders, but has been discontinued for depression.

Rolipram

This compound is thought to stimulate the synthesis and release of norepinephrine into the synapse and to uniquely affect the intracellular response of the receptor. In several trials it has been as effective as other antidepressants but has not demonstrated a specific advantage. More studies will be necessary to demonstrate that it warrants approval by the FDA.

Roxindole

Roxindole acts on dopamine and on serotonin, which accounts for its antidepressant effects as well as for its ability to decrease depression and lack of energy in schizophrenics. It is not quite clear just what Roxindole does to dopamine (whether it increases or decreases it), but it seems to have antidepressant activity. It is in active clinical trial as an anti-depressant in the United States.

S-Adenosyl-L-Methionine (SAMe)

SAMe is naturally present in all living cells, and has been investigated in a large number of disease states, including depression, Alzheimer's dementia, Parkinson's disease, HIV, liver disease, osteoarthritis, and coronary artery disease.

Twelve of thirteen controlled studies found SAMe better than placebo, and nineteen studies comparing it to a prescription antidepressant found it equal. What is clearly needed is a large, carefully designed, SAMe versus SSRI versus placebo-controlled study run by a neutral organization, such as the National Institute of Mental Health, similar to the one by Richard Shelton, et al., on St. John's Wort.

Because SAMe is an over-the-counter supplement, most insurance plans do not pay for it, and an independent laboratory (Consumerlab.com) found that only seven of the thirteen brands contained the amount of SAMe advertised on the label.

Substance P

Substance P is a naturally occurring neurotransmitter located in the brain and gastrointestinal tract that increases after acute stress, and was found to be elevated in the cerebrospinal fluid of depressed patients. Receptors called the neurokinin (NK) receptors are the targets for substance P, and a number of drugs are being developed to block NK in the hope they will have antidepressant and other effects. One of them failed to exceed placebo (MK-869), and research on it has stopped, but a second (Compound A) is in phase III clinical trials. A number of other NK blockers are also being tested (CP-122721, GW-597599, R-673, and TAK-637) for the treatment of depression, anxiety, irritable bowel syndrome, chemotherapy-induced nausea, and urinary incontinence. So far, several of these have equaled SSRIs and exceeded placebos, but after ten years of research, none have proven clearly more effective than drugs we now have. Perhaps this is due to one theory of the action of NK blockers, which is on norepinephrine and serotonin, the same ultimate targets.

Sulpride (Dogmatil)

Sulpride has been used as an antipsychotic in Europe for years, and is also officially recognized in low doses as an antidepressant in France. There are no plans for its release in the United States.

Tianeptine

The unusual and interesting thing about this drug is that it is the opposite of an SSRI, which means it enhances rather than inhibits serotonin reuptake from the synapse. I mentioned this reduction of the intrasynaptic concentration of serotonin earlier, when I referred to kicking the synapse. If there is an explanation for what is happening in the gap between brain cells, it remains to be discovered.

Tianeptine is officially available only in France. The drug needs more research. In one controlled study of 265 anxious, dysthymic patients, Tianeptine was as effective as Elavil. In a published report on depressed alcoholics, it also equaled Elavil.

Tianeptine has no cardiovascular or older tricyclic-like side effects. Its most common side effects are vomiting, nausea, irritability, anxiety, and insomnia. There are currently no plans to release it in the United States.

Transcranial Magnetic Stimulation (TMS)

Repeated powerful magnetic pulses applied to the scalp produce a current in the brain. Each group of pulses lasts several seconds and the complete treatment ten to twenty minutes. About three weeks of daily treatment is needed to improve mood symptoms, and it is unknown how long the effects will last. Preliminary reports find it may be effective in depression and relatively safe. In comparative studies with electroconvulsive therapy (ECT), ECT proved more effective. TMS produces a seizure as an occasional side effect, whereas ECT is designed to do so. Furthermore, ECT requires general anesthesia and the induction of skeletal muscle paralysis, whereas TMS patients remain awake, have no memory loss, and as soon as the treatment is over can resume their daily routines without supervision. The most serious side effect of TMS in 1 to 2 percent of the patients is unintentional induction of a seizure. Other adverse effects are scalp pain at the site of the stimulation, headaches, and the need for ear plugs to prevent auditory damage. If efficacy can be fully established (more research is needed), then TMS would be preferable to ECT.

Transdermal Selegiline

Originally approved for use in Parkinson's disease as Eldepryl at doses of 5 to 10 mg per day, to be an effective antidepressant it requires oral administration of 20 to 60 mg per day. This higher dose makes a restricted diet necessary in order to avoid hypertensive crises. Given as a skin patch (EMSAM), it does not involve the gastrointestinal tract, and thus markedly diminishes the chance of food interactions. The patch in doses of 20 to 30 mg lasts twenty-four hours, and must be applied daily. The only side effects seem to be rash and occasional burning under the patch. It is expected to be released soon.

Vagus Nerve Stimulation (VNS)

VNS therapy is delivered by a pacemaker-like device implanted on the chest, and conducted by wires to the left vagus nerve. It is now used for epilepsy. Studies in severe, nonpsychotic, treatment-resistant patients are in preliminary stages.

Vestra (Reboxetine)

Vestra (reboxetine) is available throughout Europe and is a specific norepinehrine reuptake inhibitor (SNRI), which in 2000 was ready to be approved by the FDA for release in the United States as an antidepressant. Unfortunately, the drug has not proven to be consistently more effective than placebo in American trials, and four years later remains unavailable.

The marketing machine was all prepared, announcing that norepinephrine-disordered depressions made sufferers fatigued, pleasureless, slowed down, and caused them to sleep too much. Furthermore, it was announced, Vestra had a unique effect on social functioning, and a scale was devised to prove it. Drs. Stuart Montgomery and Alan F. Shatzberg proclaimed in 1998 in the *Journal of Clinical Psychiatry* that Vestra had "differential effects on social functioning compared to the SSRIs."

What to Do Until the Next Antidepressant Breakthrough

There you have it—the twenty-four drugs I have chosen to mention, some serious contenders for release in the United States, others theoretically interesting, some so you will know what your friends and relatives abroad are taking. I have chosen to leave out many others because they seem weak, toxic, or dull copies of what we already have. I am reminded of how forty years ago the great Swiss psychiatrist Roland Kuhn, working with a slightly modified form of Thorazine, which he expected to be an antipsychotic, had the clarity of vision to observe what he did not expect to see, and thus found Tofranil, the first tricyclic antidepressant. With all our progress, no antidepressant has proven more effective than this first one. It is clear that our diagnostic tools still need to be refined, as do the medications we use to treat what we diagnose. Many dedicated psychiatric researchers are occupied in doing just that.

But until the next significant breakthrough, depression sufferers have the presently available modern antidepressants described in this book. If you are truly lucky, they will completely cure you. If, like most patients, you are complicated and not totally cured, you at least have a chance of receiving some very good help in your efforts to get control of your feelings and your life, so that you will be able to function in a full and meaningful way. Who knows what miracle medication will come along next year, genetically engineered to root out the elusive depressive gene. Somehow I suspect humans do not work that way, and that our machine requires more than a drug. It requires love and useful activity of which we can be proud, and the identification of something worth living for. It takes more than Prozac to make a full life.

Appendix:
How to Read Your
Doctor's Prescription

In this day of mega-drugstores and long lines, it makes sense to know how to read your doctor's prescription and to check to make sure the name of the medication is legible before you leave the office.

Abbreviation	Latin Phrase	English
Ad lib	ad libitum	at will; as it pleases
b.i.d.	bis in die	twice a day
t.i.d.	ter in die	three times a day
q.i.d.	quater in die	four times a day
q.d.	quaque die	every day
o.h.	omni hora	every hour
ind.	in dies	daily
quoted.	quotidie	daily

Abbreviation	Latin Phrase	English
alt. dieb.	Alternis diebus	on alternate days
q.h.	quaque hora	every hour
h.s.	hor a somni	at bedtime
a.c.	ante cibum	before a meal
p.c.	post cibum	after a meal
m.et.n.	mane et nocte	morning and night
p.r.n.	pro re nata	as occasion arises
s.o.s.	si opus sit	if necessary
Rx	recipe	take
Sig.	Signetur	let it be labeled
d.	da	give, administer
c.	cum	with
s.	sine	without
c.	circa	about, approximately
q.l.	quantum libet	as much as desired
q.s.	quantum satis	as much as is sufficient

Bibliography

Depression and Its Treatment

Akiskal, H. S. 1984. The interface of chronic depression with personality and anxiety disorders. *Psychopharmocology Bulletin* 20:393–98.

American Psychiatric Association. Practice guideline for major depressive disorder in adults. 1993. *American Journal of Psychiatry* 150 (No. 4, suppl.).

Brown, W. A., and Harrison, W. 1995. Are patients who are intolerant to one selective serotonin reuptake inhibitor intolerant to another? *Journal of Clinical Psychiatry* 56:30–34.

Coryell, W., Scheftner, W., Keller, M., et al. 1993. The enduring psychosocial consequences of mania and depression. *American Journal of Psychiatry* 150:720–27.

The Cross-National Collaborative Group. 1992. The changing rate of major depression. *Journal of the American Medical Association* 268:3098–3105.

DeVane, C. L. 1994. Pharmacogenetics and drug metabolism of newer antidepressant agents. *Journal of Clinical Psychiatry* 55 (12, suppl.):38–45.

Donovan, S. J., and Roose, S. P. 1995. Medication use during psychoanalysis: A survey. *Journal of Clinical Psychiatry* 56:177–78.

Dubovsky, S. L., and Thomas, M. 1995. Serotonergic mechanisms and current and future psychiatric practice. *Journal of Clinical Psychiatry* 56 (suppl. 2):38–48.

Hays, R. D., Wells, K. B., Sherbourne, D. C., et al. 1995. Functioning and well-being outcomes of patients with depression compared with chronic medical illness. *Archives of General Psychiatry* 52:11–19.

Hirschfeld, R. M. A. 1994. Guidelines for the long-term treatment of depression. *Journal of Clinical Psychiatry* 55 (12, suppl.):61–69.

Judd, L. L. 1994. Social phobia: A clinical overview. *Journal of Clinical Psychiatry* 55 (6, suppl.):5–9.

Keller, M. B., and Hanks, D. L. 1994. The natural history and heterogeneity of depressive disorders: Implications for rational antidepressant therapy. *Journal of Clinical Psychiatry* 55 (9, suppl. A):25–31.

———, Klerman, G. L., Lavori, P. W., et al. 1982. Treatment received by depressed patients. *Journal of the American Medical Association* 248:1848–55.

———, Lavori, P. W., Mueller, T. I., et al. 1992. Time to recovery, chronicity, and levels of psychopathology in major depression. *Archives of General Psychiatry* 49:809–16.

Kocsis, J. H., Croughan, J. L., Katz, M. M., et al. 1990. Response to treatment with antidepressants of patients with severe or moderate nonpsychotic depression and of patients with psychotic depression. *American Journal of Psychiatry* 147:621–24.

Kupfer, D. J. 1993. Management of recurrent depressions. *Journal of Clinical Psychiatry* 54 (2, suppl.): 29–33.

———, Frank, E., Perel, J. M., et al. 1992. Five-year outcome for maintenance therapies in recurrent depression. *Archives of General Psychiatry* 49:769–73.

Leonard, B. E. 1993. The comparative pharmacology of new anti-depressants. *Journal of Clinical Psychiatry* 54 (suppl.):3–15.

Liebowitz, M. R. 1989. Antidepressants in panic disorders. *British Journal of Psychiatry* 155 (suppl.):46–52.

McTavish, D., and Benfield, P. 1990. Clomipramine: An overview of its pharmacological properties and a review of its therapeutic use in obsessive-compulsive disorder and panic disorder. *Drugs* 39:136–53.

Nemeroff, C. B. 1994. Evolutionary trends in the pharmacothera-peutic management of depression. *Journal of Clinical Psychiatry* 55 (12, suppl.):3–15.

Preskorn, S. H. 1994. Antidepressant drug selection: Criteria and options. *Journal of Clinical Psychiatry* 55 (9, suppl. A):6–22.

———. 1993. Pharmacokinetics of antidepressants: Why and how they are relevant to treatment. *Journal of Clinical Psychiatry* 54 (9, suppl.):14–34.

———, and Burke, M. 1992. Somatic therapy for major depressive disorder: Selection of an antidepressant. *Journal of Clinical Psychiatry* 53 (9, suppl.):5–18.

Regier, D. A., Hirschfield, R. M. A., Goodwin, F. K., et al. 1988. The NIMH depression awareness, recognition, and treatment pro-gram: Structure, aims, and scientific basis. *American Journal of Psychiatry* 145:1351–57.

Weinberger, D. R. 1993. SPECT imaging in psychiatry: Introduction and overview. *Journal of Clinical Psychiatry* 54 (11, suppl.):3–5.

Weissman, M. M., Prusoff, B. A., Dimascio, A., et al. 1979. The effi-cacy of drugs and psychotherapy in the treatment of acute depres-sive episodes. *American Journal of Psychiatry* 136:555–58.

Wells, K. B., Stewart, A. S., Hays, R. D., et al. 1989. The functioning and well-being of depressed patients. *Journal of the American Medical Association* 262:914–19.

Fluoxetine (Prozac)

Bowden, C. L., Schatzberg, A. F., Rosenbaum, A., et al. 1993. Fluoxetine and desipramine in major depressive disorder. *Journal of Clinical Psychopharmacology* 13:305–10.

De Klerk, E. Patient complaining with enteric-coating weekly fluoxetine during continuation treatment of major depressive disorder. *Journal of Clinical Psychiatry* 62 (suppl. 22):43–57.

Fava, M., Rappe, S. M., Pava, J. A., et al. 1995. Relapse in patients on long-term fluoxetine treatment: Response to increased fluoxetine dose. *Journal of Clinical Psychiatry* 56:52–55.

———, and Rosenbaum, J. F. 1991. Suicidality and fluoxetine: Is there a relationship? *Journal of Clinical Psychiatry* 52:108–11.

Fluoxetine—a new specific serotonin reuptake inhibitor in major depressive disorder. 1985. *Journal of Clinical Psychiatry* 46 (3, sec. 2).

Gram, L. F. 1994. Fluoxetine. *New England Journal of Medicine* 17:1354–61.

Kramer, P. D. 1993. *Listening to Prozac.* New York: Viking.

Miner, C. M., Brown, E. B. Gonzales, J. S., et al. 2002. Switching patients from daily citalopram, paroxetine, or sertraline to once-weekly fluoxetine in the maintenance of response for depression. *Journal of Clinical Psychiatry* 63:232–40.

Montgomery, S. A., Dufour, H., Brion, S., et al. 1988. The prophylactic efficacy of fluoxetine in unipolar depression. *British Journal of Psychiatry* 153 (suppl. 3):69–76.

Pande, A., and Sayler, M. 1993. Severity of depression and response to fluoxetine. *International Clinical Psychopharmocology* 8:243–45.

Pearlstein, T. B., and Stone, A. B. 1994. Long-term fluoxetine treatment of late luteal phase dysphoric disorder. *Journal of Clinical Psychiatry* 55:332–35.

Pigott, T. A., Pato, M. T., Bernstein, S. E., et al. 1990. Controlled comparisons of clomipramine and fluoxetine in the treatment of obsessive-compulsive disorder. *Archives of General Psychiatry* 47:926–32.

Rickels, K., Amsterdam, J. D., and Avallone, M. F. 1986. Fluoxetine in major depression: A controlled study. *Current Therapeutic Research* 39:559–63.

Roose, S. P., Glassman, A. H., Attia, E., et al. 1994. Comparative efficacy of selective serotonin reuptake inhibitors and tricyclics in the treatment of mania. *American Journal of Psychiatry* 151:1735–39.

Salzman, C., Wolfson, A. N., Schatzberg, A., et al. 1995. Effect of fluoxetine on anger in symptomatic volunteers with borderline personality disorder. *Journal of Clinical Psychopharmacology* 15:23–29.

Stone, A. B., Pearlstein, T. B., and Brown, W. A. 1991. Fluoxetine in the treatment of late luteal phase dysphoric disorder. *Journal of Clinical Psychiatry* 52:290–93.

Wernicke, J. F., Dunlop, S. R., Dornseif, B. E., et al. 1987. Fixed-dose fluoxetine therapy for depression. *Psychopharmacology Bulletin* 23:164–68.

Sertraline (Zoloft)

Aguglia, E., Casacchia, M., Cassano, G. B., et al. 1993. Double-blind study of the efficacy and safety of sertraline and fluoxetine [Prozac] in major depression. *International Clinical Psychopharmacology* 8:197–202.

Bennie, E. H., Mullin, J. M., and Martindale, J. J. 1995. A double-blind multicenter trial comparing sertraline and fluoxetine in outpatients with major depression. *Journal of Clinical Psychiatry* 56:229–37.

Chouinard, G. 1992. Sertraline in the treatment of obsessive compulsive disorder: Two double-blind, placebo-controlled studies. *International Clinical Psychopharmacology* 7 (2, suppl.): 37–41.

Cole, J. O. 1992. New directions in antidepressant therapy: A review of sertraline, a unique serotonin reuptake inhibitor. *Journal of Clinical Psychiatry* 53:333–40.

Doogan, D. P., and Caillard, V. 1992. Sertraline in the prevention of depression. *British Journal of Psychiatry* 160:217–22.

Fisher, S., Kent, T., and Bryant, S. 1995. Postmarketing surveillance by patient self-monitoring: Preliminary data for sertraline versus fluoxetine [Prozac]. *Journal of Clinical Psychiatry* 56:288–96.

Murdoch, D., and McTavish, D. 1992. Sertraline: A review of its pharmacodynamic and pharmacokinetic properties and therapeutic potential in depression and obsessive-compulsive disorder. *Drugs* 44:604–24.

Reimherr, F. W., Chouinard, G., Cohn, C. K., et al. 1990. Antidepressant efficacy of sertraline: A double-blind placebo and amitriptyline-controlled, multicenter comparison study in outpatients with major depression. *Journal of Clinical Psychiatry* 51 (12, suppl. B):18–27.

Yonkers, K. A., Halbreich, V., Freeman, E., et al. 1997. Symptomatic improvement of premenstrual dysphoric disorder with sertraline (Zoloft) treatment: a randomized controlled trial. *Journal of the American Medical Association* 278:983–88.

Paroxetine (Paxil)

Ayd, F. J. 1993. Paroxetine: A new selective serotonin reuptake inhibitor. *International Drug Therapy Newsletter* 28 (2):5–12.

Claghorn, J. L. 1992. The safety and efficacy of paroxetine compared with placebo in a double-blind trial of depressed outpatients. *Journal of Clinical Psychiatry* 53 (2, suppl.):33–35.

Cohn, J. B., and Wilcox, C. S. 1992. Paroxetine in major depression: A double-blind trial with imipramine and placebo. *Journal of Clinical Psychiatry* 53 (2, suppl.):52–56.

De Wilde, J., Spiers, R., Mertens, C., et al. 1993. A double-blind, comparative, multicentre study comparing paroxetine with fluoxetine in depressed patients. *Acta Psychiatrica Scandinavica* 87:141–45.

Dunbar, G. C., Cohn, J. B., Fabre, L. F., et al. 1991. A comparison of paroxetine, imipramine [Tofranil], and placebo in depressed out-patients. *British Journal of Psychiatry* 159:394–98.

Eric, L. 1991. A prospective, double-blind, comparative, multicentre study of paroxetine and placebo in preventing recurrent major depressive episodes [abstract]. *Biological Psychiatry* 29 (11 S): 254S–55S.

Fabre, L. F. 1992. A six-week, double-blind trial of paroxetine, imipramine, and placebo in depressed outpatients. *Journal of Clinical Psychiatry* 53 (2, suppl.):40–43.

Feighner, J. P., and Boyer, W. F. 1992. Paroxetine in the treatment of depression: A comparison with imipramine and placebo. *Journal of Clinical Psychiatry* (2, suppl.):44–47.

Gilmor, M. L., Owens, M. J., and Nemeroff, C. B. 2002. Inhibition of norepinephrine uptake in patients with major depression treated with paroxetine. *American Journal of Psychiatry* 159:1702–10.

Golden, R. N., Nemeroff, C. B., McSorley, P., et al. 2002. Efficacy and tolerability of controlled-release and immediate-release paroxetine in the treatment of depression. *Journal of Clinical Psychiatry* 63:577–84.

Kiev, A. 1992. A double-blind, placebo-controlled study of paroxetine in depressed outpatients. *Journal of Clinical Psychiatry* 53 (suppl.):27–29.

Kreider, M. S., Bushnell, W. D., Oakes, R., et al. 1995. A double-blind, randomized study to provide safety information on switching fluoxetine-treated patients to paroxetine without an intervening washout period. *Journal of Clinical Psychiatry* 56:142–45.

Nemeroff, C. B. 1993. Paroxetine: An overview of the efficacy and safety of a new selective serotonin reuptake inhibitor in the treatment of depression. *Journal of Clinical Psychopharmacology* 13 (6, suppl. 2):10S–17S.

Rickels, K., Amsterdam, J., Clary, C., et al. 1992. The efficacy and safety of paroxetine compared with placebo in outpatients with major depression. *Journal of Clinical Psychiatry* 53 (2, suppl.):30–32.

Shrivastava, R. K., Shrivastava, S. H. P., Overweg, N., et al. 1992. A double-blind comparison of paroxetine, imipramine, and placebo in major depression. *Journal of Clinical Psychiatry* 53 (2, suppl.): 48–51.

Smith, W. T., and Glaudin, V. 1992. A placebo-controlled trial of paroxetine in the treatment of major depression. *Journal of Clinical Psychiatry* 53: (2, suppl.):36–39.

Stuppaeck, C. H., Geretsegger, C., and Whitworth, A. B. 1994. A multicenter double-blind trial of paroxetine versus amitriptyline in depressed outpatients. *Journal of Clinical Psychopharmacology* 14:241–46.

Tignol, J. 1993. A double-blind, randomized, fluoxetine-controlled, multicenter study of paroxetine in the treatment of depression. *Journal of Clinical Psychopharmacology* 13 (6, suppl. 2):18S–22S.

Fluvoxamine (Luvox)

Benfield, P., and Ward, A. 1986. Fluvoxamine: A review of its pharmacodynamic and pharmacokinetic properties and therapeutic efficacy in depressive illness. *Drugs* 32:313–34.

Burton, S. W. 1991. A review of fluvoxamine and its uses in depression. *International Clinical Psychopharmacology* (suppl. 3):1–17; discussion, 17–21.

Conti, L., Dell'osso, L., Re, F., et al. 1988. Fluvoxamine maleate: Double-blind clinical trial vs. placebo in hospitalized depressed patients. *Current Therapeutic Research* 43:468–80.

McDougle, C. J., Goodman, W. K., Leckman, J. F., et al. 1993. The efficacy of fluvoxamine in obsessive-compulsive disorder: Effects of comorbid chronic tic disorder. *Journal of Clinical Psychopharmacology* 13:354–58.

Mendlewicz, J. 1992. Efficacy of fluvoxamine in severe depression. *Drugs* 43 (suppl. 2):32–37; discussion, 37–39.

Montgomery, S. A., and Manceaux, A. 1992. Fluvoxamine in the treatment of obsessive-compulsive disorder. *International Clinical Psychopharmacology* (suppl. 1):5–9.

Wilde, M. I., Plosker, G. L., and Benfield, P. 1993. Fluvoxamine: An updated review of its pharmacology and therapeutic use in depressive illness. *Drugs* 46 (5):895–924.

Citalopram (Celexa)

Danish University Antidepressant Group. 1986. Citalopram (Celexa): clinical effect profile in comparison with clomipramine: A controlled multicenter study. *Psychopharmacology* 90:131–38.

Glassman, A. H. 1997. Citalopram (Celexa) toxicity. *Lancet* 350:818.

Lexapro (Escitalopram)

Burke, W. J., Gergel, I., and Bose, A. 2002. Fixed-dose trial of the single-isomer SSRI escitalopram in depressed outpatients. *Journal of Clinical Psychiatry* 63(4):331–36.

Gorman, J. M., Korotzer, A., and Su, G. 2002. Efficacy of escitalopram and citalopram in the treatment of major depressive disorder: Pooled analysis of placebo-controlled trials. *CNS Spectrums* 7 (suppl. 1):40–44.

Owens, M. J., and Rosenbaum, J. F. 2002. Escitalopram: A second-generation SSRI. *CNS Spectrums* 7 (suppl. 1):34–39.

Bupropion (Wellbutrin)

Clinical management of depression: Bupropion: An update. 1993. *Journal of Clinical Psychiatry*, monograph 11 (1).

Bodkin, J. A., Lasser, R. A., Wines, J. D., et al. 1997. Combining serotonin reuptake inhibitors and bupropion (Wellbutrin) in partial responders to antidepressant monotherapy. *Journal of Clinical Psychiatry* 58:137–145.

Davidson, J. 1989. Seizures and bupropion: A review. *Journal of Clinical Psychiatry* 50:256–61.

Feighner, J. P., Gardner, E. A., Johnston, J. A., et al. 1991. Double-blind comparison of bupropion and fluoxetine [Prozac] in depressed outpatients. *Journal of Clinical Psychiatry* 52:329–35.

Gardner, E. A., and Johnston, J. A. 1985. Bupropion: An antidepressant without sexual pathophysiological action. *Journal of Clinical Psychopharmacology* 5:24–29.

Hurt, R. D., Sachs, D. P. L., Glover, E. D., et al. 1997. A comparison of sustained-release bupropion (Zyban) and placebo for smoking cessation. *New England Journal of Medicine* 337:1195–1202.

Kavolussi, R. J., Segraves, R. T., Hughes, A. R., et al. 1997. Double-blind comparison of bupropion (Wellbutrin) sustained release and sertraline in depressed outpatients. *Journal of Clinical Psychiatry* 58:532–37.

Mendels, J., Amin, M. M., Chouinard, G., et al. 1983. A comparative study of bupropion and amitriptyline in depressed outpatients. *Journal of Clinical Psychiatry* 44:118–20.

Merideth, C. H., and Feighner, J. P. 1983. The use of bupropion in hospitalized depressed patients. *Journal of Clinical Psychiatry* 44:85–87.

Modell, J. G., Katholi, C. R., Modell, J. D., et al. 1997. Comparative sexual side effects of bupropion (Wellbutrin), fluoxetine (Prozac), paroxetine (Paxil), and sertraline (Zoloft). *Clinical Pharmacological Therapeutics* 61:476–87.

Pitts, W. M.; Fann, W. E., Halaris, A. E., et al. 1983. Bupropion in depression: A tricenter placebo-controlled study. *Journal of Clinical Psychiatry* 44:95–100.

Preskorn, S. H. 1991. Should bupropion dosage be adjusted based upon therapeutic drug monitoring? *Psychopharmacology Bulletin* 27:637–43.

Walker, P. W., Cole, J. O., Gardner, E. A., et al. 1993. Improvement in fluoxetine-associated sexual dysfunction in patients switched to bupropion. *Journal of Clinical Psychiatry* 54:459–65.

Weisler, R. H:, Johnston, J. A., Lineberry, C. G., et al. 1994. Comparison of bupropion and trazodone for the treatment of major depression. *Journal of Clinical Psychopharmacology* 14:170–79.

Zarate, C. A., Tohen, M., Baraibar, G., et al. 1995. Prescribing trends of antidepressants in bipolar depression. *Journal of Clinical Psychiatry* 56:260–64.

Venlafaxine (Effexor)

Boyd, I. W. 1998. Venlafaxine (Effexor) withdrawal reactions. *Medical Journal of Australia* 169:91–92.

Clerc, G. E., Ruimy, P., and Verdeau-Pailles, J. 1994. A double-blind comparison of venlafaxine and fluoxetine [Prozac] in patients hospitalized for major depression and melancholia. *International Clinical Psychopharmacology* 9:139–43.

Cunningham, L. A., Borison, R. L., Carman, J. S., et al. 1994. A comparison of venlafaxine, trazodone, and placebo in major depression. *Journal of Clinical Psychopharmacology* 14:99–106.

Derivan, A., Entsuah, R., Rudolph, R., et al. Early response to venlafaxine hydrochloride, a novel antidepressant. Proceedings of the 145th annual meeting of the American Psychiatric Association, May 2–7, 1992, Washington, D.C., pp. 82–83.

Feighner, J. P. 1994. The role of venlafaxine in rational antidepressant therapy. *Journal of Clinical Psychiatry* 55 (9, suppl. A):62–68.

Guelfi, J. D., White, C., Hackett, D., et al. 1995. Effectiveness of venlafaxine in patients hospitalized for major depression and melancholia. *Journal of Clinical Psychiatry* 56:450–58.

Khan, A., Fabre, L. F., and Rudolph, R. R. 1991. Venlafaxine in depressed outpatients. *Psychopharmacology Bulletin* 27 (2):141–44.

Mendels, J., Johnston, R., Mattes, J., et al. 1993. Efficacy and safety of b.i.d. [twice-daily] doses of venlafaxine in a dose-response study. *Psychopharmacology Bulletin* 29 (2):169–74.

Montgomery, S. A. 1993. Venlafaxine: A new dimension in antidepressant pharmacotherapy. *Journal of Clinical Psychiatry* 54:119–26.

Nierenberg, A. A., Feighner, J. P., Rudolph, R. R., et al. 1994. Venlafaxine for treatment-resistant depression. *Neuropsychopharmacology* 10 (pt. 2):85S.

Schweizer, E., Feighner, J., Mandos, L. A., et al. 1994. Comparison of venlafaxine and imipramine in the acute treatment of major depression in outpatients. *Journal of Clinical Psychiatry* 55:104–8.

————, Weise, C., Clary, C., et al. 1991. Placebo-controlled trial of venlafaxine for the treatment of major depression. *Journal of Clinical Psychopharmacology* 11 (4):233–36.

Shrivastava, R. K., Cohn, C., Crowder, J., et al. 1994. Long-term safety and clinical acceptability of venlafaxine and imipramine [Tofranil] in outpatients with major depression. *Journal of Clinical Psychopharmacology* 14:322–29.

Silverstone, P. H., and Ravindran, A. 1999. Once-daily venlafaxine (Effexor) extended release (XR) compared with fluoxetine (Prozac) in outpatients with depression and anxiety. *Journal of Clinical Psychiatry* 60:22–28.

The Venlafaxine French Inpatient Study Group. Clerc, G. E., et al. 1994. A double-blind comparison of venlafaxine and fluoxetine in patients hospitalized for major depression and melancholia. *International Clinical Psychopharmacology* 9 (3):139–43.

Nefazodone (Serzone)

Anton, S., Robinson, D., Roberts, D., et al. 1994. Long-term treatment with nefazodone. *Psychopharmacology Bulletin* 30:165–69.

Feighner, J. P., Pambakian, R., Fowler, R. C., et al. 1989. A comparison of nefazodone, imipramine, and placebo in patients with moderate to severe depression. *Psychopharmacology Bulletin* 25:219–21.

Fontaine, R., Ontiveros, A., Elie, R., et al. 1994. A double-blind comparison of nefazodone, imipramine, and placebo in major depression. *Journal of Clinical Psychiatry* 55:234–41.

————, Ontiveros, A., Faludi, G., et al. 1991. A study of nefazodone, imipramine, and placebo in depressed outpatients. *Biological Psychiatry* 29:3–38.

Preskorn, S. H. 1995. Comparison of the tolerability of bupropion [Wellbutrin], fluoxetine [Prozac], imipramine [Tofranil], nefazodone [Serzone], paroxetine [Paxil], sertraline [Zoloft], and venlafaxine [Effexor]. *Journal of Clinical Psychiatry* 56 (suppl. 6): 12–21.

Rickels, K., Robinson, D. S., Schweizer, E., et al. 1995. Nefazodone: Aspects of efficacy. *Journal of Clinical Psychiatry* 56 (suppl. 6): 43–46.

———, Schweizer, E., Clary, C., et al. 1994. Nefazodone and imipramine in major depression: A placebo-controlled trial. *British Journal of Psychiatry* 164:802–5.

Sharpley, A. L., Walsh, A. E. S., Cowen, P. J. 1992. Nefazodone—a novel antidepressant—may increase REM sleep. *Biological Psychiatry* 31:1070–73.

Taylor, D. P., Carter, R. B., Eison, A. S., et al. 1995. Pharmacology and neurochemistry of nefazodone, a novel antidepressant drug. *Journal of Clinical Psychiatry* 56 (suppl. 6):3–11.

Weise, C., Fox, I., Clary, C., et al. 1991. Nefazodone in the treatment of outpatient major depression. *Biological Psychiatry* 29:3–33.

Mirtazapine (Remeron)

Bremner, J. D. 1995. A double-blind comparison of org 3770 [Remeron], amitriptyline, and placebo in major depression. *Journal of Clinical Psychiatry* 56:519–25.

deBoer, Th. 1996. The pharmacologic profile of mirtazapine [Remeron]. *Journal of Clinical Psychiatry* 57 (suppl 4):19–25.

Fawcett, J., and Barkin, R. L. 1998. A meta-analysis of eight randomized, double-blind, controlled clinical trials of mirtazapine (Remeron) for the treatment of patients with major depression and symptoms of anxiety. *Journal of Clinical Psychiatry* 59:123–27.

Richou, H., Ruimy, P., Charbaut, J., et al. 1995. A multicenter, double-blind, clomipramine-controlled efficacy and safety study of org 3770 [Remeron]. *Human Psychopharmacology* 10:263–71.

Stimmel G. L., Sussman, N., and Wingard, P. 1997. Mirtazapine (Remeron) safety and tolerability: Analysis of the clinical trials database. *Primary Psychiatry* 4:82–91.

Wheatly, D. P., van Moffaert, M., Timmerman, L., et al., and the mirtazapine (Remeron)-fluoxetine (Prozac) study group. 1998.

Mirtazapine (Remeron): Efficacy and tolerability in comparison with fluoxetine in patients with moderate to severe major depressive disorder. *Journal of Clinical Psychiatry* 59:306–12.

Zivkov, M., and DeJongh, G. D. 1995. Org 3770 [Remeron] versus amitriptyline: A 6-week randomized double-blind multicentre trial in hospitalized depressed patients. *Human Psychopharmacology* 10: 173–80.

Zivkov, M., Roes, K. C. B., and Pols, A. G. 1995. Efficacy of org 3770 [Remeron] vs amitriptyline in patients with major depressive disorder: A meta-analysis. *Human Psychopharmacology* 10 (suppl 2): S135–S145.

Reboxetine (Vestra)

Burrows, G. D., Maguire, K. P., and Norman, T. R., 1998. Antidepressant efficacy and tolerability of the selective norepinephrine reuptake inhibitor reboxetine: A review. *Journal of Clinical Psychiatry* 59 (suppl 14):4–7.

Healy, D. 1998. Reboxetine, fluoxetine (Prozac) and social functioning as an outcome measure in antidepressant trials: Implications. *Primary Care Psychiatry* 4 (2):81–89.

Patient selection and antidepressant therapy with reboxetine, a new selective norepinephrine reuptake inhibitor. 1998. *Journal of Clinical Psychiatry* 59 (suppl. 14):3–29.

Versiani, M., Lembit, M., Gaszner, P., et al. 1999. Reboxetine, a unique selective NRI, prevents relapse and recurrence in long-term treatment of major depressive disorder. *Journal of Clinical Psychiatry* 60:400–6.

Duloxetine

Detke, M. J., Lu, Y., Goldstein, D. J., et al. 2002. Duloxetine, 60 mg once daily, for major depressive disorder: A randomized double-blind placebo-controlled trial. *Journal of Clinical Psychiatry* 63: 308–15.

Goldstein, D., Bitter, L., Lu, Y., et al. 2002. Duloxetine in the treatment of depression: A double-blind, placebo-controlled comparison with paroxetine. *European Psychiatry* 17 (suppl. 1):98.

Side Effects

Sexual

Ashton, A. K., and Rosen, R. C. 1998. Bupropion (Wellbutrin) as an antidote for serotonin reuptake inhibitor–induced sexual dysfunction. *Journal of Clinical Psychiatry* 59:112–15.

Balon, R., Yeragani, V. K., Pohl, R., et al. 1993. Sexual dysfunction during antidepressant treatment. *Journal of Clinical Psychiatry* 54:209–12.

Feiger, A., Kiev, A., Shrivastava, R. K., et al. 1996. Nefazodone versus sertraline [Zoloft] in outpatients with major depression: Focus on efficacy, tolerability, and effects on sexual function and satisfaction. *Journal of Clinical Psychiatry* 57 (suppl. 2):53–62.

Gitlin, M. J. 1994. Psychotropic medications and their effects on sexual function: Diagnosis, biology, and treatment approaches. *Journal of Clinical Psychiatry* 55:406–13.

Goldstein, I., Lue, T. F., Padma-Nathan, H., et al. 1998. Oral sildenafil (Viagra) in the treatment of erectile dysfunction. *New England Journal of Medicine* 338:1397–1404.

Hollander, E., and McCarley, A. 1992. Yohimbine treatment of sexual side effects induced by serotonin reuptake blockers. *Journal of Clinical Psychiatry* 53:207–9.

Hopkins, H. S. 1992. Antidotes for antidepressant-induced sexual dysfunction. In Gelenberg, A. G., ed., *Biological Therapies in Psychiatry* 15:33–36.

Jacobsen, F. M. 1992. Fluoxetine-induced sexual dysfunction and an open trial of yohimbine. *Journal of Clinical Psychiatry* 53:119–22.

Nurnberg, H. G., Lauriello, M. D., Hensley, P. L., et al. 1999. Sildenafil (Viagra) for iatrogenic serotonergic antidepressant medication–induced sexual dysfunction in four patients. *Journal of Clinical Psychiatry* 60(1):33–35.

Seizures

Rosenstein, D. L., Nelson, J. C., and Jacobs, S. C. 1993. Seizures associated with antidepressants: A review. *Journal of Clinical Psychiatry* 54:289–99.

Withdrawal

Ellison, J. M. 1994. SSRI withdrawal buzz. *Journal of Clinical Psychiatry* 55:544–45.

Zajecka, J., Tracy, K. A., and Mitchell, S. 1997. Discontinuation symptoms after treatment with serotonin reuptake inhibitors: A literature review. *Journal of Clinical Psychiatry* 58:1–7.

General

McElroy, S. L., Keck, P. E., and Friedman, L. M. 1995. Minimizing and managing antidepressant side effects. *Journal of Clinical Psychiatry* 56 (suppl. 2):49–55.

Nelson, J. C. 1994. Are the SSRIs really better tolerated than the TCAs for treatment of major depression? *Psychiatric Annuals* 24:628–31.

Nierenberg, A. A., and Cole, J. O. 1991. Antidepressant adverse drug reactions. *Journal of Clinical Psychiatry* 52 (suppl.):40–47.

Serotonin Syndrome

Sternbach, H. 1991. The serotonin syndrome. *American Journal of Psychiatry* 148:705–13.

Mania

Peet, M. 1994. Induction of mania with selective serotonin reuptake inhibitors and tricyclic antidepressants. *British Journal of Psychiatry* 164:549–50.

Stoll, A. L., Mayer, P. V., Kolbrener, M., et al. 1994. Antidepressant-associated mania: A controlled comparison with spontaneous mania. *American Journal of Psychiatry* 151:1642–45.

Antidepressants During Pregnancy and Lactation

Goldstein, D. J., Corbin, L. A., and Sundell, K. L. 1997. Effects of first trimester fluoxetine (Prozac) exposure on the newborn. *Obstetrics and Gynecology* 89:713–18.

Kulin, N. A., Pastuszak, A., and Sage, S. R., et al. 1998. Pregnancy outcome following maternal use of the new selective serotonin reuptake inhibitors: A prospective controlled multicenter study. *Journal of the American Medical Association* 279:609–10.

Wisner, K. L., Perel, J. M., and Findling, R. L. 1996. Antidepressant treatment during breastfeeding. *American Journal of Psychiatry* 153:1132–37.

Bipolar Disorder

American Psychiatric Association. 1994. Practice guideline for the treatment of patients with bipolar disorder. *American Journal of Psychiatry* 151 (12, suppl.).

Bowden, C. L. 1995. Predictors of response to divalproex [Depakote] and lithium. *Journal of Clinical Psychiatry* 56 (suppl. 3):25–30.

———. 1998. Key treatment studies of lithium in manic-depressive illness: Efficacy and side effects. *Journal of Clinical Psychiatry* 5a (suppl. 6):13–19.

———, and McElroy, S. L. 1995. History of the development of valproate [Depakene and others] for treatment of bipolar disorder. *Journal of Clinical Psychiatry* 56 (suppl. 3):3–5.

Carlson, G. A., and Goodwin, F. K. 1973. The stages of mania. *Archives of General Psychiatry* 28:221–28.

Freeman, M. P., and Stoll, A. L. 1998. Mood stabilizer combinations: A review of safety and efficacy. *American Journal of Psychiatry* 155:12–21.

Goodwin, F. K., and Jamison, K. R. 1990. Medical treatment of manic episodes. In Goodwin, F. K., and Jamison, K. R., eds.,

Manic Depressive Illness, pp. 603–29. New York: Oxford University Press.

Isojarvi, J. I. T., Laatikainen, T. J., and Pakarinen, A. J., et al. 1993. Polycystic ovaries and hyperandrogenism in women taking valproate for epilepsy. *New England Journal of Medicine* 329:1383–88.

Kusumakar, V., and Yatham, L. N. 1997. Lamotrigine treatment of rapid cycling bipolar disorder. *American Journal of Psychiatry* 154:1171–72.

Marangell, L. B., and Yudofsky, S. C. 1995. Developments in the treatment of bipolar disorder. *Primary Psychiatry* 2 (6):32–41.

McElroy, S. L., Soutullo, C. A., and Keck, P. E., et al. 1997. A pilot trial of adjunctive gabapentin in the treatment of bipolar disorder. *Annals of Clinical Psychiatry* 9:99–103.

Small, J. G., Klapper, M. H., Milstein, V., et al. 1991. Carbamazepine [Tegretol] compared with lithium in the treatment of mania. *Archives of General Psychiatry* 48:915–21.

Solomon, D. A., Keitner, G. I., Miller, I. W., et al. 1995. Course of illness and maintenance treatments for patients with bipolar disorder. *Journal of Clinical Psychiatry* 56:5–13.

Benzodiazepines

Bruce, S. E., Vasile, R. G., Goisman, R. M., et al. 2003. Are benzodiazepines still the medication of choice for patients with panic disorder with or without agoraphobia? *American Journal of Psychiatry* 160:1432–38.

Greenblatt, D. J., Shader, R. I., and Abernethy, D. R. 1983. Current status of benzodiazepines. Part 1 of 2. *New England Journal of Medicine* 309:354–59.

Greenblatt, D. J., Shader, R. I., and Abernethy, D. R. 1983. Current status of benzodiazepines. Part 2 of 2. *New England Journal of Medicine* 309:410–15.

Noyes, R., Burrows, G. D., Reich, J. H., et al. 1996. Diazepam versus alprazolam for the treatment of panic disorders. *Journal of Clinical Psychiatry* 57:349–55.

Piper, A. 1995. Addiction to benzodiazepines—how common? *Archives of Family Medicine* 4:964–70.

Rickels, K., Downing, R., Schweizer, E., et al. 1993. Antidepressants for the treatment of generalized anxiety disorder: A placebo-controlled comparison of imipramine, trazodone, and diazepam. *Archives of General Psychiatry* 50:884–95.

Roache, J. D., and Meisch, R. A. 1995. Findings from self-administration research on the addiction potential of benzodiazepines. *Psychiatric Annals* 25:153–57.

Romach, M., Busto, U., Somer, G., et al. 1995. Clinical aspects of chronic use of alprazolam and lorazepam. *American Journal of Psychiatry* 152:1161–70.

Salzman, C., for Task Force on Benzodiazepine Dependency, American Psychiatric Association. 1990. Benzodiazepine dependence, toxicity and abuse: A task force report of the American Psychiatric Association, Washington, D.C. American Psychiatric Association.

Uhlenhuth, E. H., DeWit, H., Balter, M. B., et al. 1988. Risks and benefits of long-term benzodiazepine use. *Journal of Clinical Psychopharmacology* 8:161–67.

Insomnia

Jindal, R. D., Buysse, D. J., and Thase, M. E. 2004. Maintenance treatment of insomnia: What can we learn from the depression literature? *American Journal of Psychiatry* 161:19–24.

Kupfer, D. J., and Reynolds, C. F., III. 1997. Management of insomnia. *New England Journal of Medicine* 336:341–46.

Nowell, P. D., Mazumdar, S., Buysse, D. J., et al. 1997. Benzodiazepines and zolpidem for chronic insomnia: A meta-analysis of treatment efficacy. *Journal of the American Medical Association* 278:2170–77.

Treatment-Resistant Depression

Klein, R. G., and Wender, P. 1995. The role of methylphenidate [Ritalin] in psychiatry. *Archives of General Psychiatry* 52:429–33.

Management of patients who are nonresponders to or nontolerators of initial antidepressant therapy. 1992. *Journal of Clinical Psychiatry*, monograph 10 (1).

Nelson, J. C. 1993. Combined treatment strategies in psychiatry. *Journal of Clinical Psychiatry* 54 (suppl.):42–49.

Nemeroff, C. B. 1991. Augmentation regimens for depression. *Journal of Clinical Psychiatry* 52 (5, suppl):21–27.

Phillips, K. A., and Nierenberg, A. A. 1994. The assessment and treatment of refractory depression. *Journal of Clinical Psychiatry* 55 (2, suppl.):20–26.

Zajecka, J. M., Jeffriess, H., and Fawcett, J. 1995. The efficacy of fluoxetine [Prozac] combined with a heterocyclic antidepressant in treatment-resistant depression: A retrospective analysis. *Journal of Clinical Psychiatry* 56:338–43.

Provigil (Modafinil)

DeBattista, C., Doghramji, K., Menza, M. A., et al. 2003. Adjunct modafinil for the short-term treatment of fatigue and sleepiness in patients with major depressive disorder: A preliminary double-blind placebo-controlled study. *Journal of Clinical Psychiatry* 64:1057–64.

Strattera (Atomoxetine)

Spencer, T., Heiligenstein, J. H., Biederman, J., et al. 2002. Results from 2 proof-of-concept, placebo-controlled studies of atomoxetine in children with attention-deficit/hyperactivity disorder. *Journal of Clinical Psychiatry* 63:1140–47.

Herbal Medicines

Almeida, J. C., and Grimsley, E. W. 1996. Coma form the health food store: Interaction between kava and alprazolam (Xanax). *Annals of Internal Medicine* 125:940–41.

Lecrubier, Y., Clerc, G., Didi, R., et al. 2002. Efficacy of St. John's Wort extract WS 5570 in major depression: A double-blind, placebo-controlled trial. *American Journal of Psychiatry* 159: 1361–66.

Linde, K., Ramirez, G., Mulrow, C. D., et al. 1996. St. John's Wort for depression—an overview and meta-analysis of randomized clinical trials. *British Medical Journal* 313:253–58.

Shelton, R. C., Keller, M. H. Gelenberg, A., et al. 2001. Effectiveness of St. John's Wort in major depression: A randomized controlled trial. *Journal of the American Medical Association* 285:1978–86.

Wong, A. H. C., Smith, M., and Boon, H. S. 1998. Herbal remedies in psychiatric practice. *Archives of General Psychiatry* 55:1033–44.

Substance P

Kramer, M. S., Cutler, N., Feighner, J., et al. 1998. Distinct mechanism for antidepressant activity by blockade of central substance P receptors. *Science* 281:1640–45.

The Future and the Available Unproven

Gepirone ER

Feiger, A. D. 1996. A double-blind comparison of gepirone extended release, imipramine, and placebo in the treatment of outpatient major depression. *Psychopharmacology Bulletin* 32:659–65.

Mifepristone (RU-486, the Abortion Pill)

Belanoff, J., Flores, B., Kalezhan, M., et al. 2001. Rapid reversal of psychotic major depression using mifepristone. *Journal of Clinical Psychopharmacology* 21:516–21.

Omega-3 Fatty Acids

Nemets, B., Stahl, Z., and Belmaker, R. H. 2002. Addition of omega-3 fatty acid to maintenance medication treatment for recurrent unipolar depressive disorder. *American Journal of Psychiatry* 159: 477–79.

Stoll, A. L., Severus, W. E., Freeman, M. P., et al. 1999. Omega-3 fatty acids in bipolar disorder: A preliminary double-blind, placebo-controlled trial. *Archives of General Psychiatry* 56:407–12.

S-Adenosyl-L-Methionine (SAMe)

Bressa, G. M. 1994. S-adenosyl-L-methionine (SAMe) as antidepressant: Meta-analysis of clinical studies. *Acta Neurologica Scandinavica Supplementum* 154:7–14.

Transcranial Magnetic Stimulation

George, M. S., Wasserman, E. M., Kimbrell, T. A., et al. 1997. Mood improvement following daily left prefrontal repetitive transcranial magnetic stimulation in patients with depression: a placebo-controlled cross-over trial. *American Journal of Psychiatry* 154:1752–56.

Gershon, A. A., Dannon, P. N., and Grunhaus, L. 2003. Transcranial magnetic stimulation in the treatment of depression. *American Journal of Psychiatry* 160:835–45.

Janicak, P. G., Krasuski, J., Beedle, B., et al. 1999. Transcranial magnetic stimulation for neuropsychiatric disorders. *Psychiatric Times* 16:2:56–63.

Transdermal Selegiline

Bodkin, J. A., and Amsterdam, J. D. 2002. Transdermal selegiline in major depression: A double-blind, placebo-controlled, parallel-group study in outpatients. *American Journal of Psychiatry* 159: 1869–75.

Bodkin, J. A., and Kwon, A. E. 2001. Selegiline and other atypical monoamine oxidase inhibitors in depression. *Psychiatric Annals* 31:385–91.

Vagus Nerve Stimulation (VNS)

George, M., et al. 2000. Vagus nerve stimulation: A new tool for brain research and therapy. *Biological Psychiatry* 47:287–95.

General Reference

American Psychiatric Association: Diagnostic and Statistical Manual of Mental Disorders. 2000. 4th ed. Text revision. Washington, D.C.: American Psychiatric Association.

Appleton, W. S. 1991. *The Fifth Psychoactive Drug Usage Guide.* Memphis: Physicians Postgraduate Press.

———. 1988. *Practical Clinical Psychopharmacology.* 3d ed. Baltimore: Williams and Wilkins.

Beck, A. T. 1967. *Depression: Causes and Treatment.* Philadelphia: University of Pennsylvania Press.

Bloom, F. E., and Kupfer, D. J., eds. 1995. *Psychopharmacology: The Fourth Generation of Progress.* New York: Raven Press.

Hales, R. E., Yudofsky, S. C., and Talbott, J. A. 1999. *The American Psychiatric Press Textbook of Psychiatry.* 3d ed. Washington, D.C.: American Psychiatric Press.

Healy, D. 1997. *The Antidepressant Era.* Cambridge: Harvard University Press.

Hyman, S. E., and Nestler, E. J. 1993. *The Molecular Foundations of Psychiatry.* Washington, D.C.: American Psychiatric Press.

Janicak, P. G., Davis, J. M., Preskorn, S. H., and Ayd, F. J. 1997. *Principles and Practice of Psychopharmacotherapy*, 2nd ed. Baltimore: Williams and Wilkins.

Schatzberg, A. F., Cole, J. O., and DeBattista, C. 2003. *Manual of Clinical Psychopharmacology*, 4th ed. Washington, D.C.: American Psychiatric Press.

————, and Nemeroff, C. B., eds. 2004. *The American Psychiatric Press Textbook of Psychopharmacology*, 3d ed. Washington, D.C.: American Psychiatric Press.

Stein, D. J., and Hollander, E., eds. 2002. *The American Psychiatric Publishing Textbook of Anxiety Disorders*. Washington, D.C.: American Psychiatric Publishing.

Index